THE *ITALIAN DIET*

FOR weight loss Cookbook

More than 300 HEALTHY Mediterranean Recipes for Weight Loss and stay FIT! Tone your Body before SUMMER and Maintain your Perfect Weight with The Best Diet Overall!

3 BOOKS IN 1

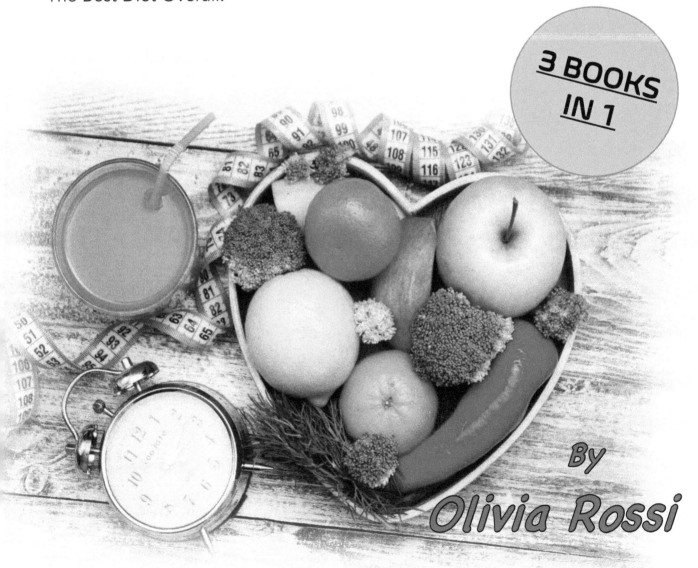

By

Olivia Rossi

Table of Contents

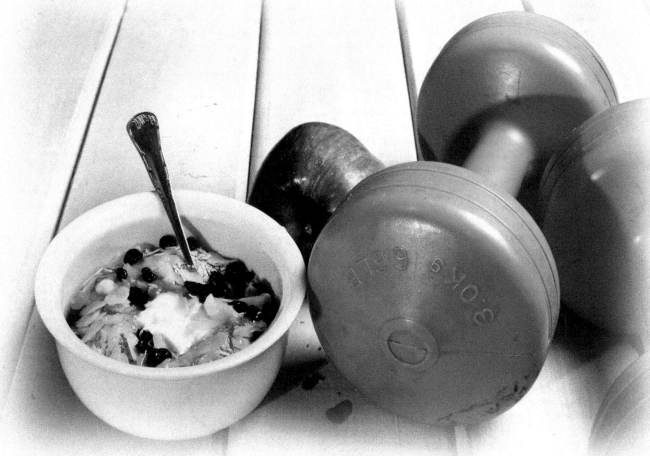

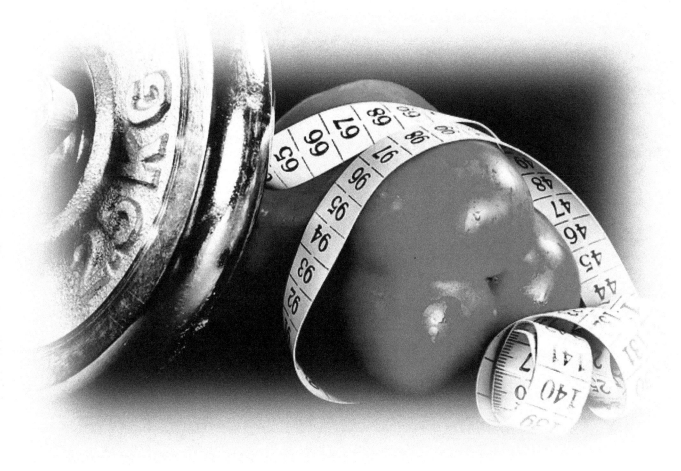

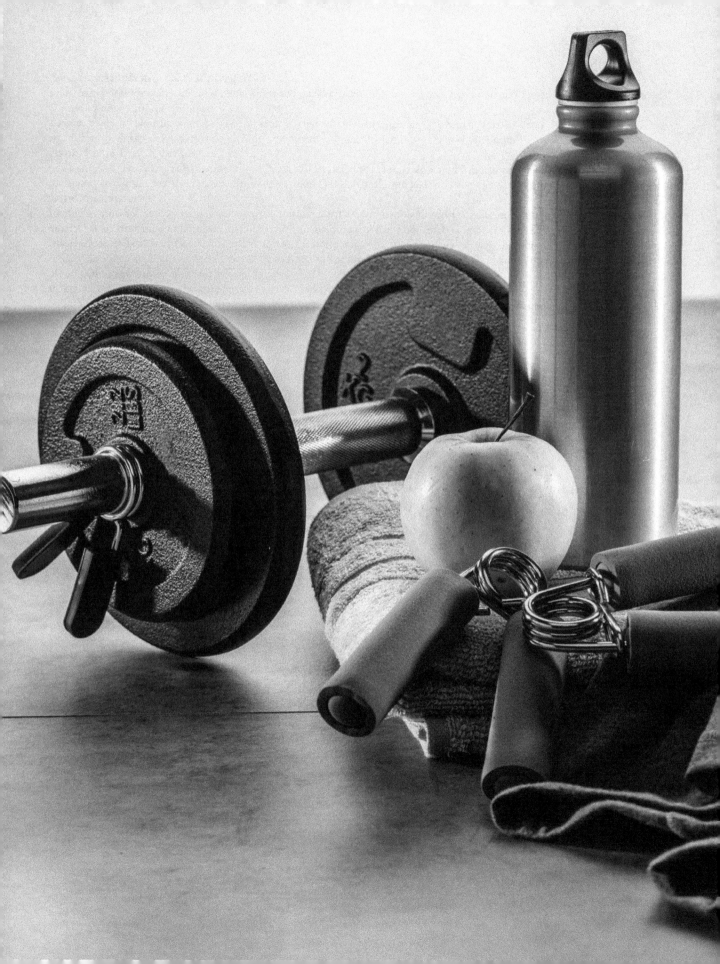

Introduction

Everyone knows Italian Cuisine: it is one of the most delicious and Healthy diet in the world! Everybody can follow Italian Diet: **children**, **older people**, **beginners**, **women**, and **men**! And, what is no better to have the right amount of nutrients while eating delicious meals?

Did you know it? **Scientists discovered that to have a healthy body and lose weight you must eat well. For eating well, people must eat high-quality foods and the right amount of nutrients in each moment of the day.**
But, does a specific diet that help you to have the right amount with tasty meals exist? Yes: The Italian Diet!
"The Italian Diet for Lose Weight *Cookbook*" was born for all **people** who want to have a fantastic lunch or dinners **while maintaining their body FIT**, or while wanting to lose weight! Indeed, this cookbook is a collection of 3 of my favorite books: "The Italian Diet for Beginners *Cookbook*", "The Italian Diet for One *Cookbook*", and "The Italian Diet for Men *Cookbook*": **the perfect combination you need to lose weight and stay FIT!**

You can choose many recipes with the best Italian ingredients such as:
- Cereals: bread, pasta, pizza
- Legumes: green beans, chickpeas, beans
- Proteins: milk, cheese, red meat, fish, light meat, seafood, nuts, extra virgin olive oil
- Fibers and vitamins: all of vegetables and fruits
Note - If you want to delight yourself: Add raw extra virgin olive oil to your food for the best experience ever! In the Italian Diet, it is important the quality of foods: foods must be fresh and, if possible, must be cultivated in Italy.

Do you want to know The Best 320 Italian Recipes for your Fitness?

LET'S GO Together!

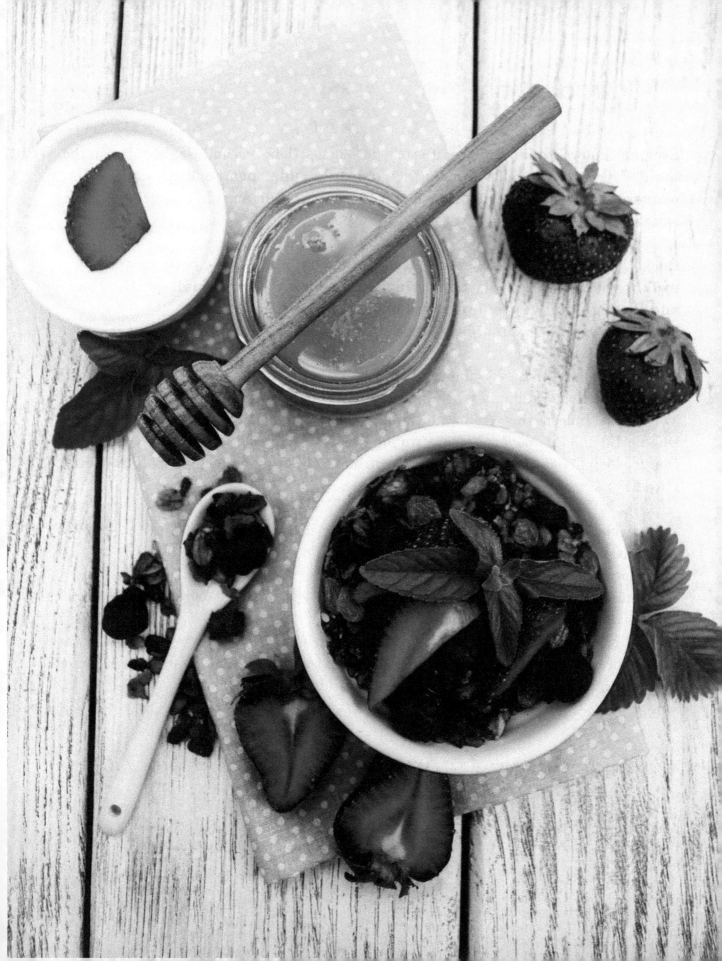

Chapter 1. BREAKFAST AND SNACKS

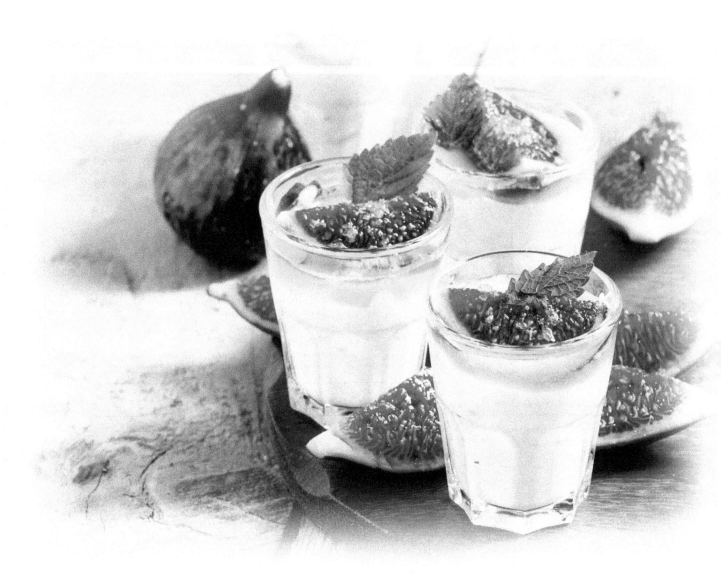

1) SPECIAL CAULIFLOWER FRITTERS AND HUMMUS

	Cooking Time: 15 Minutes	Servings: 4

Ingredients:

- ✓ 2 (15 oz) cans chickpeas, divided
- ✓ 2 1/2 tbsp olive oil, divided, plus more for frying
- ✓ 1 cup onion, chopped, about 1/2 a small onion
- ✓ 2 tbsp garlic, minced
- ✓ 2 cups cauliflower, cut into small pieces, about 1/2 a large head
- ✓ 1/2 tsp salt
- ✓ black pepper
- ✓ Topping:
- ✓ Hummus, of choice
- ✓ Green onion, diced

Directions:

- ❖ Preheat oven to 400°F
- ❖ Rinse and drain 1 can of the chickpeas, place them on a paper towel to dry off well
- ❖ Then place the chickpeas into a large bowl, removing the loose skins that come off, and toss with 1 tbsp of olive oil, spread the chickpeas onto a large pan (being careful not to over-crowd them) and sprinkle with salt and pepper
- ❖ Bake for 20 minutes, then stir, and then bake an additional 5-10 minutes until very crispy
- ❖ Once the chickpeas are roasted, transfer them to a large food processor and process until broken down and crumble - Don't over process them and turn it into flour, as you need to have some texture. Place the mixture into a small bowl, set aside
- ❖ In a large pan over medium-high heat, add the remaining 1 1/2 tbsp of olive oil
- ❖ Once heated, add in the onion and garlic, cook until lightly golden brown, about 2 minutes. Then add in the chopped cauliflower, cook for an additional 2 minutes, until the cauliflower is golden
- ❖ Turn the heat down to low and cover the pan, cook until the cauliflower is fork tender and the onions are golden brown and caramelized, stirring often, about 3-5 minutes
- ❖ Transfer the cauliflower mixture to the food processor, drain and rinse the remaining can of chickpeas and add them into the food processor, along with the salt and a pinch of pepper. Blend until smooth, and the mixture starts to ball, stop to scrape down the sides as needed
- ❖ Transfer the cauliflower mixture into a large bowl and add in 1/2 cup of the roasted chickpea crumbs (you won't use all of the crumbs, but it is easier to break them down when you have a larger amount.), stir until well combined
- ❖ In a large bowl over medium heat, add in enough oil to lightly cover the bottom of a large pan
- ❖ Working in batches, cook the patties until golden brown, about 2-3 minutes, flip and cook again
- ❖ Distribute among the container, placing parchment paper in between the fritters. Store in the fridge for 2-3 days
- ❖ To Serve: Heat through in the oven at 350F for 5-8 minutes. Top with hummus, green onion and enjoy!
- ❖ Recipe Notes: Don't add too much oil while frying the fritter or they will end up soggy. Use only enough to cover the pan. Use a fork while frying and resist the urge to flip them every minute to see if they are golden

Nutrition: Calories:333;Total Carbohydrates: 45g;Total Fat: 13g;Protein: 14g

2) ITALIAN BREAKFAST SAUSAGE AND NEW POTATOES WITH VEGETABLES

	Cooking Time: 30 Minutes	**Servings: 4**
✓ 1 lbs sweet Italian sausage links, sliced on the bias (diagonal) ✓ 2 cups baby potatoes, halved ✓ 2 cups broccoli florets ✓ 1 cup onions cut to 1-inch chunks ✓ 2 cups small mushrooms -half or quarter the large ones for uniform size	✓ 1 cup baby carrots ✓ 2 tbsp olive oil ✓ 1/2 tsp garlic powder ✓ 1/2 tsp Italian seasoning ✓ 1 tsp salt ✓ 1/2 tsp pepper	❖ Preheat the oven to 400 degrees F ❖ In a large bowl, add the baby potatoes, broccoli florets, onions, small mushrooms, and baby carrots ❖ Add in the olive oil, salt, pepper, garlic powder and Italian seasoning and toss to evenly coat ❖ Spread the vegetables onto a sheet pan in one even layer ❖ Arrange the sausage slices on the pan over the vegetables ❖ Bake for 30 minutes – make sure to sake halfway through to prevent sticking ❖ Allow to cool ❖ Distribute the Italian sausages and vegetables among the containers and store in the fridge for 2-3 days ❖ To Serve: Reheat in the microwave for 1-2 minutes, or until heated through and enjoy! ❖ Recipe Notes: If you would like crispier potatoes, place them on the pan and bake for 15 minutes before adding the other ingredients to the pan.

3) GREEK QUINOA BREAKFAST BOWL

	Cooking Time: 20 Minutes	**Servings: 6**
✓ 12 eggs ✓ ¼ cup plain Greek yogurt ✓ 1 tsp onion powder ✓ 1 tsp granulated garlic ✓ ½ tsp salt ✓ ½ tsp pepper	✓ 1 tsp olive oil ✓ 1 (5 oz) bag baby spinach ✓ 1 pint cherry tomatoes, halved ✓ 1 cup feta cheese ✓ 2 cups cooked quinoa	❖ In a large bowl whisk together eggs, Greek yogurt, onion powder, granulated garlic, salt, and pepper, set aside ❖ In a large skillet, heat olive oil and add spinach, cook the spinach until it is slightly wilted, about 3-4 minutes. Add in cherry tomatoes, cook until tomatoes are softened, 4 minutes. Stir in egg mixture and cook until the eggs are set, about 7-9 minutes, stir in the eggs as they cook to scramble ❖ Once the eggs have set stir in the feta and quinoa, cook until heated through. Distribute evenly among the containers, store for 2-3 days ❖ To serve: Reheat in the microwave for 30 seconds to 1 minute or heated through

4) EGG, HAM AND CHEESE SANDWICHES IN THE FREEZER

	Cooking Time: 20 Minutes	**Servings: 6**
✓ Cooking spray or oil to grease the baking dish ✓ 7 large eggs ✓ ½ cup low-fat (2%) milk ✓ ½ tsp garlic powder ✓ ½ tsp onion powder	✓ 1 tbsp Dijon mustard ✓ ½ tsp honey ✓ 6 whole-wheat English muffins ✓ 6 slices thinly sliced prosciutto ✓ 6 slices Swiss cheese	❖ Preheat the oven to 375°F. Lightly oil or spray an 8-by--inch glass or ceramic baking dish with cooking spray. ❖ In a large bowl, whisk together the eggs, milk, garlic powder, and onion powder. Pour the mixture into the baking dish and bake for minutes, until the eggs are set and no longer jiggling. Cool. ❖ While the eggs are baking, mix the mustard and honey in a small bowl. Lay out the English muffin halves to start assembly. ❖ When the eggs are cool, use a biscuit cutter or drinking glass about the same size as the English muffin diameter to cut 6 egg circles. Divide the leftover egg scraps evenly to be added to each sandwich. ❖ Spread ½ tsp of honey mustard on each of the bottom English muffin halves. Top each with 1 slice of prosciutto, 1 egg circle and scraps, 1 slice of cheese, and the top half of the muffin. ❖ Wrap each sandwich tightly in foil. ❖

5) TAHINI EGG SALAD AND PITA		
Cooking Time: 12 Minutes		**Servings: 4**

✓ 4 large eggs ✓ ¼ cup freshly chopped dill ✓ 1 tbsp plus 1 tsp unsalted tahini	✓ 2 tsp freshly squeezed lemon juice ✓ ⅛ tsp kosher salt ✓ 4 whole-wheat pitas, quartered	❖ Place the eggs in a saucepan and cover with water. Bring the water to a boil. As soon as the water starts to boil, place a lid on the pan and turn the heat off. Set a timer for minutes. ❖ When the timer goes off, drain the hot water and run cold water over the eggs to cool. ❖ When the eggs are cool, peel them, place the yolks in a medium bowl, and mash them with a fork. Then chop the egg whites. ❖ Add the chopped egg whites, dill, tahini, lemon juice (to taste), and salt to the bowl, and mix to combine. ❖ Place a heaping ⅓ cup of egg salad in each of 4 containers. Place the pita in 4 separate containers or resealable bags so that the bread does not get soggy. ❖ STORAGE: Store covered containers in the refrigerator for up to 5 days.

6) MANGO STRAWBERRY- GREEN SMOOTHIE		
Cooking Time: 10 Minutes		**Servings: 2**

✓ 1½ cups low-fat (2%) milk ✓ 2 cups packed baby spinach leaves ✓ ½ cup sliced Persian or English cucumber, skin on	✓ ⅔ cup frozen strawberries ✓ ⅔ cup frozen mango chunks ✓ 1 medium very ripe banana, sliced (about ⅔ cup) ✓ ½ small avocado ✓ 1 tsp honey	❖ Place the milk, spinach, cucumber, strawberries, mango, banana, and avocado in a blender. ❖ Blend until smooth and taste. If the smoothie isn't sweet enough, add the honey. ❖ Distribute the smoothie between 2 to-go cups. ❖ STORAGE: Store smoothie cups in the refrigerator for up to 3 days.

7) BREAKFAST TACO SCRAMBLE		
Cooking Time: 1 Hour 25 Minutes		**Servings: 4**

✓ 8 large eggs, beaten ✓ 1/4 tsp seasoning salt ✓ 1 lb 99% lean ground turkey ✓ 2 tbsp Greek seasoning ✓ 1/2 small onion, minced ✓ 2 tbsp bell pepper, minced ✓ 4 oz. can tomato sauce ✓ 1/4 cup water	✓ 1/4 cup chopped scallions or cilantro, for topping ✓ For the potatoes: ✓ 12 (1 lb) baby gold or red potatoes, quartered ✓ 4 tsp olive oil ✓ 3/4 tsp salt ✓ 1/2 tsp garlic powder ✓ fresh black pepper, to taste	❖ In a large bowl, beat the eggs, season with seasoning salt ❖ Preheat the oven to 4 degrees F ❖ Spray a 9x12 or large oval casserole dish with cooking oil ❖ Add the potatoes 1 tbsp oil, 3/tsp salt, garlic powder and black pepper and toss to coat ❖ Bake for 4minutes to 1 hour, tossing every 15 minutes ❖ In the meantime, brown the turkey in a large skillet over medium heat, breaking it up while it cooks ❖ Once no longer pink, add in the Greek seasoning ❖ Add in the bell pepper, onion, tomato sauce and water, stir and cover, simmer on low for about 20 minutes ❖ Spray a different skillet with nonstick spray over medium heat ❖ Once heated, add in the eggs seasoned with 1/4 tsp of salt and scramble for 2–3 minutes, or cook until it sets ❖ Distribute 3/4 cup turkey and 2/3 cup eggs and divide the potatoes in each storage container, store for 3-4 days ❖ To Serve: Reheat in the microwave for 1-minute (until 90% heated through) top with shredded cheese if desired, and chopped scallions

Nutrition: (¼ of a the scramble): Calories:450;Total Fat: 19g;Total Carbs: 24.5g;Fiber: 4g;Protein: 46g

8) SPICED CRANBERRY TEA

	Cooking Time: 18 Minutes	Servings: 2

Ingredients:

- ✓ 1-ounce cranberries
- ✓ ½ lemon, juice, and zest
- ✓ 1 cinnamon stick
- ✓ 2 teabags
- ✓ ½ inch ginger, peeled and grated
- ✓ raw honey to taste
- ✓ 3 cups water

Directions:

- ❖ Start by adding all the Ingredients: except honey into a pot or saucepan.
- ❖ Bring to a boil and then simmer for about 115 minutes.
- ❖ Strain and serve the tea.
- ❖ Add honey or any other sweetener of your preference.
- ❖ Enjoy.

Nutrition: Calories: 38, Total Fat: 0.3g, Saturated Fat: 0.1, Cholesterol: 0 mg, Sodium: 2 mg, Total Carbohydrate: 10 g, Dietary Fiber: 4.9 g, Total Sugars: 1.1 g, Protein: 0.7 g, Vitamin D: 0 mcg, Calcium: 77 mg, Iron: 1 mg, Potassium: 110 mg

9) ZUCCHINI PUDDING

	Cooking Time: 10 Minutes	Servings: 4

Ingredients:

- ✓ 2 cups zucchini, grated
- ✓ 1/2 tsp ground cardamom
- ✓ 1/4 cup swerve
- ✓ 5 oz half and half
- ✓ 5 oz unsweetened almond milk
- ✓ Pinch of salt

Directions:

- ❖ Spray instant pot from inside with cooking spray.
- ❖ Add all ingredients into the instant pot and stir well.
- ❖ Seal pot with lid and cook on high for 10 minutes.
- ❖ Once done, allow to release pressure naturally for 10 minutes then release remaining using quick release. Remove lid.
- ❖ Stir well and serve.

Nutrition: Calories: ;Fat: 4.7 g;Carbohydrates: 18.9 g;Sugar: 16 g;Protein: 1.9 g;Cholesterol: 13 mg

10) ITALIAN STYLE BREAKFAST BURRITO

	Cooking Time: 20 Minutes	Servings: 6

Ingredients:

- ✓ 9 eggs
- ✓ 3 tbsp chopped sun-dried tomatoes
- ✓ 6 tortillas that are 10 inches
- ✓ 2 cups baby spinach
- ✓ ½ cup feta cheese
- ✓ ¾ cups of canned refried beans
- ✓ 3 tbsp sliced black olives
- ✓ Salsa, sour cream, or any other toppings you desire

Directions:

- ❖ Wash and dry your spinach.
- ❖ Grease a medium frying pan with oil or nonstick cooking spray.
- ❖ Add the eggs into the pan and cook for about 5 minutes. Make sure you stir the eggs well, so they become scrambled.
- ❖ Combine the black olives, spinach, and sun-dried tomatoes with the eggs. Stir until the ingredients are fully incorporated.
- ❖ Add the feta cheese and then set the lid on the pan so the cheese will melt quickly.
- ❖ Spoon a bit of egg mixture into the tortilla.
- ❖ Wrap the tortillas tightly.
- ❖ Wash your pan or get a new skillet. Remember to grease the pan.
- ❖ Set each tortilla into the pan and cook each side for a couple of minutes. Once they are lightly brown, remove them from the pan and allow the burritos to cool on a serving plate. Top with your favorite condiments and enjoy!
- ❖ To store the burritos, wrap them in aluminum foil and place them in the fridge. They can be stored for up to two days.

Nutrition: calories: 252, fats: grams, carbohydrates: 21 grams, protein: 14 grams

11) HEALTHY DRIED FRUIT PORRIDGE

	Cooking Time: 8 Hours	Servings: 6

✓ 2 cups steel-cut oats ✓ 1/8 tsp ground nutmeg ✓ 1 tsp vanilla ✓ 1 1/2 tsp cinnamon ✓ 1/2 cup dry apricots, chopped	✓ 1/2 cup dry cranberries, chopped ✓ 1/2 cup dates, chopped ✓ 1/2 cup raisins ✓ 8 cups of water ✓ Pinch of salt	❖ Spray instant pot from inside with cooking spray. ❖ Add all ingredients into the instant pot and stir well. ❖ Seal the pot with a lid and select slow cook mode and cook on low for 8 hours. ❖ Stir well and serve.

12) SCRAMBLED EGGS WITH PESTO SAUCE

	Cooking Time: 10 Minutes	Servings: 2

✓ 5 eggs ✓ 2 tbsp butter ✓ 2 tbsp pesto	✓ 4 tbsp milk ✓ salt to taste ✓ pepper to taste	❖ Beat the eggs into a bowl and add salt and pepper as per your taste. ❖ Then, heat a pan and add the butter, then the eggs, stirring continuously. ❖ While stirring continuously, add the pesto. ❖ Switch off the heat and quickly add the creamed milk and mix it well with eggs. ❖ Serve hot.

13) SWEET POTATOES AND SPICED MAPLE YOGURT WITH NUTS FOR BREAKFAST

	Cooking Time: 45 Minutes	Servings: 4

Ingredients: ✓ 4 red garnet sweet potatoes, about 6 inches long and 2 inches in diameter ✓ 2 cups low-fat (2%) plain Greek yogurt	✓ ¼ tsp pumpkin pie spice ✓ 1 tbsp pure maple syrup ✓ ½ cup walnut pieces	❖ Preheat the oven to 425°F. Line a sheet pan with a silicone baking mat or parchment paper. ❖ Prick the sweet potatoes in multiple places with a fork and place on the sheet pan. Bake until tender when pricked with a paring knife, 40 to 45 minutes. ❖ While the potatoes are baking, mix the yogurt, pumpkin pie spice, and maple syrup until well combined in a medium bowl. ❖ When the potatoes are cool, slice the skin down the middle vertically to open up each potato. If you'd like to eat the sweet potatoes warm, place 1 potato in each of containers and ½ cup of spiced yogurt plus 2 tbsp of walnut pieces in each of 4 other containers. If you want to eat the potatoes cold, place ½ cup of yogurt and 2 tbsp of walnuts directly on top of each of the 4 potatoes in the 4 containers.

14) BLUEBERRY AND PEACH OATMEAL

	Cooking Time: 4 Hours	Servings: 4
✓ 1 cup steel-cut oats ✓ 1/2 cup blueberries	✓ 3 1/2 cups unsweetened almond milk ✓ 7 oz can peach ✓ Pinch of salt	❖ Spray instant pot from inside with cooking spray. ❖ Add all ingredients into the instant pot and stir well. ❖ Seal the pot with a lid and select slow cook mode and cook on low for 4 hours. ❖ Stir well and serve.

Nutrition: 1;Fat: 4.5 g;Carbohydrates: 25.4 g;Sugar: 8.6 g;Protein: 3.9 g;Cholesterol: 0 mg

15) ITALIAN-STYLE VEGGIE QUICHE

	Cooking Time: 55 Minutes	Servings: 8
✓ 1/2 cup sundried tomatoes - dry or in olive oil* ✓ Boiling water ✓ 1 prepared pie crust ✓ 2 tbsp vegan butter ✓ 1 onion, diced ✓ 2 cloves garlic, minced ✓ 1 red pepper, diced ✓ 1/4 cup sliced Kalamata olives	✓ 1 tsp dried oregano ✓ 1 tsp dried parsley ✓ 1/3 cup crumbled feta cheese ✓ 4 large eggs ✓ 1 1/4 cup milk ✓ 2 cups fresh spinach or 1/2 cup frozen spinach, thawed and squeezed dry ✓ Salt, to taste ✓ Pepper, to taste ✓ 1 cup shredded cheddar cheese, divided	❖ If you're using dry sundried tomatoes - In a measure cup, add the sundried tomatoes and pour the boiling water over until just covered, allow to sit for 5 minutes or until the tomatoes are soft. The drain and chop tomatoes, set asidePreheat oven to 375 degrees F ❖ Fit a 9-inch pie plate with the prepared pie crust, then flute edges, and set aside ❖ In a skillet over medium high heat, melt the butter ❖ Add in the onion and garlic, and cook until fragrant and tender, about 3 minutes ❖ Add in the red pepper, cook for an additional 3 minutes, or until the peppers are just tender ❖ Add in the spinach, olives, oregano, and parsley, cook until the spinach is wilted (if you're using fresh) or heated through (if you're using frozen), about 5 minutes ❖ Remove the pan from heat, stir in the feta cheese and tomatoes, spoon the mixture into the prepared pie crust, spreading out evenly, set aside ❖ In a medium-sized mixing bowl, whisk together the eggs, 1/2 cup of the cheddar cheese, milk, salt, and pepper ❖ Pour this egg and cheese mixture evenly over the spinach mixture in the pie crust. Sprinkle top with the remaining cheddar cheese ❖ Bake for 50-55 minutes, or until the crust is golden brown and the egg is set. Allow to cool completely before slicing ❖ Wrap the slices in plastic wrap and then aluminum foil and place in the freezer. ❖ To Serve: Remove the aluminum foil and plastic wrap, and microwave for 2 minutes, then allow to rest for 30 seconds, enjoy! ❖ Recipe Notes: You'll find two types of sundried tomatoes available in your local grocery store—dry ones and ones packed in olive oil. Both will work for this recipe. ❖ If you decide to use dry ones, follow the directions in the recipe to reconstitute them. If you're using oil-packed sundried tomatoes, skip the first step and just remove them from the oil, chop them, and continue with the recipe.

16) SCRAMBLED EGGS ITALIAN STYLE

	Cooking Time: 10 Minutes	**Servings: 2**

✓ 1 tbsp oil ✓ 1 yellow pepper, diced ✓ 2 spring onions, sliced ✓ 8 cherry tomatoes, quartered ✓ 2 tbsp sliced black olives	✓ 1 tbsp capers ✓ 4 eggs ✓ 1/4 tsp dried oregano ✓ Black pepper ✓ Topping: ✓ Fresh parsley, to serve	❖ In a frying pan over medium heat, add the oil ❖ Once heated, add the diced pepper and chopped spring onions, cook for a few minutes, until slightly soft ❖ Add in the quartered tomatoes, olives and capers, and cook for 1 more minute ❖ Crack the eggs into the pan, immediately scramble with a spoon or spatula ❖ Sprinkle with oregano and plenty of black pepper, and stir until the eggs are fully cooked ❖ Distribute the eggs evenly into the containers, store in the fridge for 2-3 days ❖ To Serve: Reheat in the microwave for 30 seconds or in a toaster oven until warmed through

Nutrition: Calories:249;Carbs: 13g;Total Fat: 17g;Protein: 14g

17) PUDDING WITH CHIA

	Cooking Time: 15 Minutes	**Servings: 2**

Ingredients:	✓ 1 tbsp honey	Directions:
✓ ½ cup chia seeds ✓ 2 cups milk		❖ Combine and mix the chia seeds, milk, and honey in a bowl. ❖ Put the mixture in the freezer and let it set. ❖ Take the pudding out of the freezer only when you see that the pudding has thickened. ❖ Serve chilled.

18) RICE BOWLS FOR BREAKFAST

	Cooking Time: 8 Minutes	**Servings: 4**

✓ 1 cup of brown rice ✓ 1 tsp ground cinnamon ✓ 1/4 cup almonds, sliced ✓ 2 tbsp sunflower seeds	✓ 1/4 cup pecans, chopped ✓ 1/4 cup walnuts, chopped ✓ 2 cup unsweetened almond milk ✓ Pinch of salt	Directions: ❖ Spray instant pot from inside with cooking spray. ❖ Add all ingredients into the instant pot and stir well. ❖ Seal pot with lid and cook on high for 8 minutes. ❖ Once done, allow to release pressure naturally for 5 minutes then release remaining using quick release. Remove lid. ❖ Stir well and serve.

Nutrition: Calories: 291;Fat: 12 g;Carbohydrates: 40.1 g;Sugar: 0.4 g;Protein: 7.g;Cholesterol: 0 mg

19) **Quick Spinach, Feta with Egg Breakfast Quesadillas**		
	Cooking Time: 15 Minutes	**Servings: 5**
✓ 8 eggs (optional) ✓ 2 tsp olive oil ✓ 1 red bell pepper ✓ 1/2 red onion ✓ 1/4 cup milk	✓ 4 handfuls of spinach leaves ✓ 1 1/2 cup mozzarella cheese ✓ 5 sun-dried tomato tortillas ✓ 1/2 cup feta ✓ 1/4 tsp salt ✓ 1/4 tsp pepper ✓ Spray oil	❖ In a large non-stick pan over medium heat, add the olive oil ❖ Once heated, add the bell pepper and onion, cook for 4-5 minutes until soft ❖ In the meantime, whisk together the eggs, milk, salt and pepper in a bowl ❖ Add in the egg/milk mixture into the pan with peppers and onions, stirring frequently, until eggs are almost cooked through ❖ Add in the spinach and feta, fold into the eggs, stirring until spinach is wilted and eggs are cooked through ❖ Remove the eggs from heat and plate ❖ Spray a separate large non-stick pan with spray oil, and place over medium heat ❖ Add the tortilla, on one half of the tortilla, spread about ½ cup of the egg mixture ❖ Top the eggs with around ⅓ cup of shredded mozzarella cheese ❖ Fold the second half of the tortilla over, then cook for 2 minutes, or until golden brown ❖ Flip and cook for another minute until golden brown ❖ Allow the quesadilla to cool completely, divide among the container, store for 2 days or wrap in plastic wrap and foil, and freeze for up to 2 months ❖ To Serve: Reheat in oven at 375 for 3-5 minutes or until heated through

Nutrition: (1/2 quesadilla): Calories:213;Total Fat: 11g;Total Carbs: 15g;Protein: 15g

20) **BREAKFAST COBBLER**		
	Cooking Time: 12 Minutes	**Servings: 4**
✓ 2 lbs apples, cut into chunks ✓ 1 1/2 cups water ✓ 1/4 tsp nutmeg ✓ 1 1/2 tsp cinnamon	✓ 1/2 cup dry buckwheat ✓ 1/2 cup dates, chopped ✓ Pinch of ground ginger	❖ Spray instant pot from inside with cooking spray. ❖ Add all ingredients into the instant pot and stir well. ❖ Seal pot with a lid and select manual and set timer for 12 minutes. ❖ Once done, release pressure using quick release. Remove lid. ❖ Stir and serve.

21) **EGG QUINOA AND KALE BOWL**		
	Cooking Time: 5 Minutes	**Servings: 2**
✓ 1-ounce pancetta, chopped ✓ 1 bunch kale, sliced ✓ ½ cup cherry tomatoes, halved ✓ 1 tsp red wine vinegar	✓ 1 cup cooked quinoa ✓ 1 tsp olive oil ✓ 2 eggs ✓ 1/3 cup avocado, sliced ✓ sea salt or plain salt ✓ fresh black pepper	❖ Start by heating pancetta in a skillet until golden brown. Add in kale and further cook for 2 minutes. ❖ Then, stir in tomatoes, vinegar, and salt and remove from heat. ❖ Now, divide this mixture into 2 bowls, add avocado to both, and then set aside. ❖ Finally, cook both the eggs and top each bowl with an egg. ❖ Serve hot with toppings of your choice.

22) SPECIAL COCONUT BANANA MIX

	Cooking Time: 4 Minutes	**Servings: 4**

Ingredients	Ingredients	Instructions
✓ 1 cup coconut milk ✓ 1 banana ✓ 1 cup dried coconut ✓ 2 tbsp ground flax seed	✓ 3 tbsp chopped raisins ✓ ⅛ tsp nutmeg ✓ ⅛ tsp cinnamon ✓ Salt to taste	❖ Set a large skillet on the stove and set it to low heat. ❖ Chop up the banana. ❖ Pour the coconut milk, nutmeg, and cinnamon into the skillet. ❖ Pour in the ground flaxseed while stirring continuously. ❖ Add the dried coconut and banana. Mix the ingredients until combined well. Allow the mixture to simmer for 2 to 3 minutes while stirring occasionally. Set four airtight containers on the counter. ❖ Remove the pan from heat and sprinkle enough salt for your taste buds. ❖ Divide the mixture into the containers and place them into the fridge overnight. They can remain in the fridge for up to 3 days. ❖ Before you set this tasty mixture in the microwave to heat up, you need to let it thaw on the counter for a bit.

23) RASPBERRY AND LEMON MUFFINS WITH OLIVE OIL

	Cooking Time: 20 Minutes	**Servings: 12**

Ingredients	Ingredients	Instructions
✓ Cooking spray to grease baking liners ✓ 1 cup all-purpose flour ✓ 1 cup whole-wheat flour ✓ ½ cup tightly packed light brown sugar ✓ ½ tsp baking soda ✓ ½ tsp aluminum-free baking powder	✓ ⅛ tsp kosher salt ✓ 1¼ cups buttermilk ✓ 1 large egg ✓ ¼ cup extra-virgin olive oil ✓ 1 tbsp freshly squeezed lemon juice ✓ Zest of 2 lemons ✓ 1¼ cups frozen raspberries (do not thaw)	❖ Preheat the oven to 400°F and line a muffin tin with baking liners. Spray the liners lightly with cooking spray. ❖ In a large mixing bowl, whisk together the all-purpose flour, whole-wheat flour, brown sugar, baking soda, baking powder, and salt. ❖ In a medium bowl, whisk together the buttermilk, egg, oil, lemon juice, and lemon zest. ❖ Pour the wet ingredients into the dry ingredients and stir just until blended. Do not overmix. Fold in the frozen raspberries. ❖ Scoop about ¼ cup of batter into each muffin liner and bake for 20 minutes, or until the tops look browned and a paring knife comes out clean when inserted. Remove the muffins from the tin to cool. ❖ STORAGE: Store covered containers at room temperature for up to 4 days. To freeze muffins for up to 3 months, wrap them in foil and place in an airtight resealable bag.

24) EASY COUSCOUS PEARL SALAD

	Cooking Time: 10 Minutes	**Servings: 6**

Ingredients	Ingredients	Instructions
✓ lemon juice, 1 large lemon ✓ 1/3 cup extra-virgin olive oil ✓ 1 tsp dill weed ✓ 1 tsp garlic powder ✓ salt ✓ pepper ✓ 2 cups Pearl Couscous ✓ 2 tbsp extra virgin olive oil ✓ 2 cups grape tomatoes, halved ✓ water as needed	✓ 1/3 cup red onions, finely chopped ✓ ½ English cucumber, finely chopped ✓ 1 15-ounce can chickpeas ✓ 1 14-ounce can artichoke hearts, roughly chopped ✓ ½ cup pitted Kalamata olives ✓ 15-20 pieces fresh basil leaves, roughly torn and chopped ✓ 3 ounces fresh mozzarella	❖ Start by preparing the vinaigrette by mixing all Ingredients: in a bowl. Set aside. ❖ Heat olive oil in a medium-sized heavy pot over medium heat. ❖ Add couscous and cook until golden brown. ❖ Add 3 cups of boiling water and cook the couscous according to package instructions. ❖ Once done, drain in a colander and put it to the side. ❖ In a large mixing bowl, add the rest of the Ingredients: except the cheese and basil. ❖ Add the cooked couscous, basil, and mix everything well. ❖ Give the vinaigrette a gentle stir and whisk it into the couscous salad. Mix well. ❖ Adjust/add seasoning as desired. ❖ Add mozzarella cheese. ❖ Garnish with some basil. ❖ Enjoy!

25) EGG CUPS WITH TOMATO AND MUSHROOMS

		Cooking Time: 5 Minutes	Servings: 4

Ingredients	Ingredients	Directions
✓ 4 eggs ✓ 1/2 cup tomatoes, chopped ✓ 1/2 cup mushrooms, chopped ✓ 2 tbsp fresh parsley, chopped	✓ 1/4 cup half and half ✓ 1/2 cup cheddar cheese, shredded ✓ Pepper ✓ Salt	❖ In a bowl, whisk the egg with half and half, pepper, and salt. ❖ Add tomato, mushrooms, parsley, and cheese and stir well. ❖ Pour egg mixture into the four small jars and seal jars with lid. ❖ Pour 1 1/2 cups of water into the instant pot then place steamer rack in the pot. Place jars on top of the steamer rack. ❖ Seal pot with lid and cook on high for 5 minutes. ❖ Once done, release pressure using quick release. Remove lid. ❖ Serve and enjoy.

26) ITALIAN SALAD FOR BREAKFAST

		Cooking Time: 10 Minutes	Servings: 2

Ingredients	Ingredients	Directions
✓ 4 eggs (optional) ✓ 10 cups arugula ✓ 1/2 seedless cucumber, chopped ✓ 1 cup cooked quinoa, cooled ✓ 1 large avocado ✓ 1 cup natural almonds, chopped	✓ 1/2 cup mixed herbs like mint and dill, chopped ✓ 2 cups halved cherry tomatoes and/or heirloom tomatoes cut into wedges ✓ Extra virgin olive oil ✓ 1 lemon ✓ Sea salt, to taste ✓ Freshly ground black pepper, to taste	❖ Cook the eggs by soft-boiling them - Bring a pot of water to a boil, then reduce heat to a simmer. Gently lower all the eggs into water and allow them to simmer for 6 minutes. Remove the eggs from water and run cold water on top to stop the cooking, process set aside and peel when ready to use ❖ In a large bowl, combine the arugula, tomatoes, cucumber, and quinoa ❖ Divide the salad among 2 containers, store in the fridge for 2 days ❖ To Serve: Garnish with the sliced avocado and halved egg, sprinkle herbs and almonds over top. Drizzle with olive oil, season with salt and pepper, toss to combine. Season with more salt and pepper to taste, a squeeze of lemon juice, and a drizzle of olive oil

Nutrition: Calories:2;Carbs: 18g;Total Fat: 16g;Protein: 10g

27) BREAKFAST WITH CARROT OATMEAL

	Cooking Time: 10 Minutes	Servings: 2

✓ 1 cup steel-cut oats ✓ 1/2 cup raisins ✓ 1/2 tsp ground nutmeg ✓ 1/2 tsp ground cinnamon	✓ 2 carrots, grated ✓ 2 cups of water ✓ 2 cups unsweetened almond milk ✓ 1 tbsp honey	❖ Spray instant pot from inside with cooking spray. ❖ Add all ingredients into the instant pot and stir well. ❖ Seal pot with lid and cook on high for 10 minutes. ❖ Once done, release pressure using quick release. Remove lid. ❖ Stir and serve.

Nutrition: Calories: 3;Fat: 6.6 g;Carbohydrates: 73.8 g;Sugar: 33.7 g;Protein: 8.1 g;Cholesterol: 0 mg

28) ARBORIO RICE PUDDING WITH RUM AND RAISINS

	Cooking Time: 4 Hours	Servings: 2

✓ ¾ cup Arborio rice ✓ 1 can evaporated milk ✓ ½ cup raisins ✓ ¼ tsp nutmeg, grated	✓ 1½ cups water ✓ 1/3 cup sugar ✓ ¼ cup dark rum ✓ sea salt or plain salt	**Directions:** ❖ Start by mixing rum and raisins in a bowl and set aside. ❖ Then, heat the evaporated milk and water in a saucepan and then simmer. ❖ Now, add sugar and stir until dissolved. ❖ Finally, convert this milk mixture into a slow cooker and stir in rice and salt. Cook on low heat for hours. ❖ Now, stir in the raisin mixture and nutmeg and let sit for 10 minutes. ❖ Serve warm.

29) SPECIAL ITALIAN-STYLE QUINOA WITH FETA EGG MUFFINS

	Cooking Time: 30 Minutes	Servings: 12

✓ 8 eggs ✓ 1 cup cooked quinoa ✓ 1 cup crumbled feta cheese ✓ 1/4 tsp salt ✓ 2 cups baby spinach finely chopped ✓ 1/2 cup finely chopped onion	✓ 1 cup chopped or sliced tomatoes, cherry or grape tomatoes ✓ 1/2 cup chopped and pitted Kalamata olives ✓ 1 tbsp chopped fresh oregano ✓ 2 tsp high oleic sunflower oil plus optional extra for greasing muffin tins	❖ Pre-heat oven to 350 degrees F ❖ Prepare 1silicone muffin holders on a baking sheet, or grease a 12-cup muffin tin with oil, set aside ❖ In a skillet over medium heat, add the vegetable oil and onions, sauté for 2 minutes ❖ Add tomatoes, sauté for another minute, then add spinach and sauté until wilted, about 1 minute ❖ Remove from heat and stir in olives and oregano, set aside ❖ Place the eggs in a blender or mixing bowl and blend or mix until well combined ❖ Pour the eggs in to a mixing bowl (if you used a blender) then add quinoa, feta cheese, veggie mixture, and salt, and stir until well combined ❖ Pour mixture in to silicone cups or greased muffin tins, dividing equally, and bake for 30 minutes, or until eggs have set and muffins are a light golden brown ❖ Allow to cool completely ❖ Distribute among the containers, store in fridge for 2-3 days ❖ To Serve: Heat in the microwave for 30 seconds or until slightly heated through ❖ Recipe Notes: Muffins can also be eaten cold. For the quinoa, I recommend making a large batch \'7b2 cups water per each cup of dry, rinsed quinoa\'7d and saving the extra for leftovers.

Nutrition: Calories:1Total Carbohydrates: 5g;Total Fat: 7g;Protein: 6g

30) HEALTHY SALAD ZUCCHINI CABBAGE TOMATO

	Cooking Time: 20 Minutes	Servings: 4

Ingredients:

- ✓ 1 lb kale, chopped
- ✓ 2 tbsp fresh parsley, chopped
- ✓ 1 tbsp vinegar
- ✓ 1/2 cup can tomato, crushed
- ✓ 1 tsp paprika
- ✓ 1 cup zucchini, cut into cubes
- ✓ 1 cup grape tomatoes, halved
- ✓ 2 tbsp olive oil
- ✓ 1 onion, chopped
- ✓ 1 leek, sliced
- ✓ Pepper
- ✓ Salt

Directions:

- ❖ Add oil into the inner pot of instant pot and set the pot on sauté mode.
- ❖ Add leek and onion and sauté for 5 minutes.
- ❖ Add kale and remaining ingredients and stir well.
- ❖ Seal pot with lid and cook on high for 15 minutes.
- ❖ Once done, allow to release pressure naturally for 10 minutes then release remaining using quick release. Remove lid.
- ❖ Stir and serve.

Nutrition: Calories: 162;Fat: 3 g;Carbohydrates: 22.2 g;Sugar: 4.8 g;Protein: 5.2 g;Cholesterol: 0 mg

31) Bacon Brie omelette with radish salad

	Cooking Time: 10 Minutes	Servings: 6

Ingredients:

- ✓ 200 g smoked lardons
- ✓ 3 tsp olive oil, divided
- ✓ 7 ounces smoked bacon
- ✓ 6 lightly beaten eggs
- ✓ small bunch chives, snipped up
- ✓ 3½ ounces sliced brie
- ✓ 1 tsp red wine vinegar
- ✓ 1 tsp Dijon mustard
- ✓ 1 cucumber, deseeded, halved, and sliced up diagonally
- ✓ 7 ounces radish, quartered

Directions:

- ❖ Heat up the grill.
- ❖ Add 1 tsp of oil to a small pan and heat on the grill.
- ❖ Add lardons and fry them until nice and crisp.
- ❖ Drain the lardon on kitchen paper.
- ❖ Heat the remaining 2 tsp of oil in a non-sticking pan on the grill.
- ❖ Add lardons, eggs, chives, and ground pepper, and cook over low heat until semi-set.
- ❖ Carefully lay the Brie on top, and grill until it has set and is golden in color.
- ❖ Remove from pan and cut into wedges.
- ❖ Make the salad by mixing olive oil, mustard, vinegar, and seasoning in a bowl.
- ❖ Add cucumber and radish and mix well.
- ❖ Serve the salad alongside the Omelette wedges in containers.
- ❖ Enjoy!

32) OATMEAL WITH CRANBERRIES

	Cooking Time: 6 Minutes	Servings: 2

		Directions:
✓ 1/2 cup steel-cut oats	✓ 1/4 tsp vanilla	❖ Add all ingredients into the heat-safe dish and stir well.
✓ 1 cup unsweetened almond milk	✓ 1/4 cup dried cranberries	❖ Pour 1 cup of water into the instant pot then place the trivet in the pot.
✓ 1 1/2 tbsp maple syrup	✓ 1 cup of water	❖ Place dish on top of the trivet.
✓ 1/4 tsp cinnamon	✓ 1 tsp lemon zest, grated	❖ Seal pot with lid and cook on high for 6 minutes.
	✓ 1/4 cup orange juice	❖ Once done, allow to release pressure naturally for 10 minutes then release remaining using quick release. Remove lid.
		❖ Serve and enjoy.

Nutrition: Calories: 161;Fat: 3.2 g;Carbohydrates: 29.9 g;Sugar: 12.4 g;Protein: 3.4 g;Cholesterol: 0 mg

33) FIGS TOAST WITH RICOTTA CHEESE

	Cooking Time: 15 Minutes	Servings: 1

Ingredients:	✓ 1 dash cinnamon	Directions:
	✓ 2 figs (sliced)	❖ Start by mixing ricotta with honey and dash of cinnamon.
✓ 2 slices whole-wheat toast	✓ 1 tsp sesame seeds	❖ Then, spread this mixture on the toast.
✓ 1 tsp honey		❖ Now, top with fig and sesame seeds.
✓ ¼ cup ricotta (partly skimmed)		❖ Serve.

34) QUICK SPINACH, FETA WITH EGG BREAKFAST QUESADILLAS

	Cooking Time: 15 Minutes	Servings: 5

Ingredients:	✓ 4 handfuls of spinach leaves	Directions:
✓ 8 eggs (optional)	✓ 1 1/2 cup mozzarella cheese	❖ In a large non-stick pan over medium heat, add the olive oil
✓ 2 tsp olive oil	✓ 5 sun-dried tomato tortillas	❖ Once heated, add the bell pepper and onion, cook for 4-5 minutes until soft
✓ 1 red bell pepper	✓ 1/2 cup feta	❖ In the meantime, whisk together the eggs, milk, salt and pepper in a bowl
✓ 1/2 red onion	✓ 1/4 tsp salt	❖ Add in the egg/milk mixture into the pan with peppers and onions, stirring frequently, until eggs are almost cooked through
✓ 1/4 cup milk	✓ 1/4 tsp pepper	❖ Add in the spinach and feta, fold into the eggs, stirring until spinach is wilted and eggs are cooked through
	✓ Spray oil	❖ Remove the eggs from heat and plate
		❖ Spray a separate large non-stick pan with spray oil, and place over medium heat
		❖ Add the tortilla, on one half of the tortilla, spread about ½ cup of the egg mixture
		❖ Top the eggs with around ⅓ cup of shredded mozzarella cheese
		❖ Fold the second half of the tortilla over, then cook for 2 minutes, or until golden brown
		❖ Flip and cook for another minute until golden brown
		❖ Allow the quesadilla to cool completely, divide among the container, store for 2 days or wrap in plastic wrap and foil, and freeze for up to 2 months
		❖ To Serve: Reheat in oven at 375 for 3-5 minutes or until heated through

35) BREAKFAST COBBLER

Cooking Time: 12 Minutes   **Servings: 4**

Ingredients:

- ✓ 2 lbs apples, cut into chunks
- ✓ 1 1/2 cups water
- ✓ 1/4 tsp nutmeg
- ✓ 1 1/2 tsp cinnamon
- ✓ 1/2 cup dry buckwheat
- ✓ 1/2 cup dates, chopped
- ✓ Pinch of ground ginger

Directions:

- ❖ Spray instant pot from inside with cooking spray.
- ❖ Add all ingredients into the instant pot and stir well.
- ❖ Seal pot with a lid and select manual and set timer for 12 minutes.
- ❖ Once done, release pressure using quick release. Remove lid.
- ❖ Stir and serve.

Nutrition: Calories: 195;Fat: 0.9 g;Carbohydrates: 48.3 g;Sugar: 25.8 g;Protein: 3.3 g;Cholesterol: 0 mg

37) EGG QUINOA AND KALE BOWL

Cooking Time: 5 Minutes   **Servings: 2**

Ingredients:

- ✓ 1-ounce pancetta, chopped
- ✓ 1 bunch kale, sliced
- ✓ ½ cup cherry tomatoes, halved
- ✓ 1 tsp red wine vinegar
- ✓ 1 cup cooked quinoa
- ✓ 1 tsp olive oil
- ✓ 2 eggs
- ✓ 1/3 cup avocado, sliced
- ✓ sea salt or plain salt
- ✓ fresh black pepper

Directions:

- ❖ Start by heating pancetta in a skillet until golden brown. Add in kale and further cook for 2 minutes.
- ❖ Then, stir in tomatoes, vinegar, and salt and remove from heat.
- ❖ Now, divide this mixture into 2 bowls, add avocado to both, and then set aside.
- ❖ Finally, cook both the eggs and top each bowl with an egg.
- ❖ Serve hot with toppings of your choice.

38) GREEK STRAWBERRY COLD YOGURT

Cooking Time: 2-4 Hours   **Servings: 5**

Ingredients:

- ✓ 3 cups plain Greek low-fat yogurt
- ✓ 1 cup sugar
- ✓ ¼ cup lemon juice, freshly squeezed
- ✓ 2 tsp vanilla
- ✓ 1/8 tsp salt
- ✓ 1 cup strawberries, sliced

Directions:

- ❖ In a medium-sized bowl, add yogurt, lemon juice, sugar, vanilla, and salt.
- ❖ Whisk the whole mixture well.
- ❖ Freeze the yogurt mix in a 2-quart ice cream maker according to the given instructions.
- ❖ During the final minute, add the sliced strawberries.
- ❖ Transfer the yogurt to an airtight container.
- ❖ Place in the freezer for 2-4 hours.
- ❖ Remove from the freezer and allow it to stand for 5-15 minutes.
- ❖ Serve and enjoy!

Nutrition: Calories: 251, Total Fat: 0.5 g, Saturated Fat: 0.1 g, Cholesterol: 3 mg, Sodium: 130 mg, Total Carbohydrate: 48.7 g, Dietary Fiber: 0.6 g, Total Sugars: 47.3 g, Protein: 14.7 g, Vitamin D: 1 mcg, Calcium: 426 mg, Iron: 0 mg, Potassium: 62 mg

39) SPECIAL PEACH ALMOND OATMEAL

	Cooking Time: 10 Minutes	Servings: 2

✓ 1 cup unsweetened almond milk ✓ 2 cups of water	✓ 1 cup oats ✓ 2 peaches, diced ✓ Pinch of salt	❖ Spray instant pot from inside with cooking spray. ❖ Add all ingredients into the instant pot and stir well. ❖ Seal pot with a lid and select manual and set timer for 10 minutes. ❖ Once done, allow to release pressure naturally for 10 minutes then release remaining using quick release. Remove lid. Stir and serve.

40) EVERYDAY BANANA PEANUT BUTTER PUDDING

	Cooking Time: 25 Minutes	Servings: 1

✓ 2 bananas, halved ✓ ¼ cup smooth peanut butter	✓ Coconut for garnish, shredded	❖ Start by blending bananas and peanut butter in a blender and mix until smooth or desired texture obtained. ❖ Pour into a bowl and garnish with coconut if desired. Enjoy.

41) SPECIAL COCONUT BANANA MIX

	Cooking Time: 4 Minutes	Servings: 4

✓ 1 cup coconut milk ✓ 1 banana ✓ 1 cup dried coconut ✓ 2 tbsp ground flax seed	✓ 3 tbsp chopped raisins ✓ ⅛ tsp nutmeg ✓ ⅛ tsp cinnamon ✓ Salt to taste	❖ Set a large skillet on the stove and set it to low heat. ❖ Chop up the banana. ❖ Pour the coconut milk, nutmeg, and cinnamon into the skillet. ❖ Pour in the ground flaxseed while stirring continuously. ❖ Add the dried coconut and banana. Mix the ingredients until combined well. ❖ Allow the mixture to simmer for 2 to 3 minutes while stirring occasionally. ❖ Set four airtight containers on the counter. ❖ Remove the pan from heat and sprinkle enough salt for your taste buds. ❖ Divide the mixture into the containers and place them into the fridge overnight. They can remain in the fridge for up to 3 days. ❖ Before you set this tasty mixture in the microwave to heat up, you need to let it thaw on the counter for a bit.

42) RASPBERRY AND LEMON MUFFINS WITH OLIVE OIL

	Cooking Time: 20 Minutes	Servings: 12

✓ Cooking spray to grease baking liners ✓ 1 cup all-purpose flour ✓ 1 cup whole-wheat flour ✓ ½ cup tightly packed light brown sugar ✓ ½ tsp baking soda ✓ ½ tsp aluminum-free baking powder	✓ ⅛ tsp kosher salt ✓ 1¼ cups buttermilk ✓ 1 large egg ✓ ¼ cup extra-virgin olive oil ✓ 1 tbsp freshly squeezed lemon juice ✓ Zest of 2 lemons ✓ 1¼ cups frozen raspberries (do not thaw)	❖ Preheat the oven to 400°F and line a muffin tin with baking liners. Spray the liners lightly with cooking spray. ❖ In a large mixing bowl, whisk together the all-purpose flour, whole-wheat flour, brown sugar, baking soda, baking powder, and salt. ❖ In a medium bowl, whisk together the buttermilk, egg, oil, lemon juice, and lemon zest. ❖ Pour the wet ingredients into the dry ingredients and stir just until blended. Do not overmix. ❖ Fold in the frozen raspberries. ❖ Scoop about ¼ cup of batter into each muffin liner and bake for 20 minutes, or until the tops look browned and a paring knife comes out clean when inserted. Remove the muffins from the tin to cool. ❖ STORAGE: Store covered containers at room temperature for up to 4 days. To freeze muffins for up to 3 months, wrap them in foil and place in an airtight resealable bag.

43) EASY COUSCOUS PEARL SALAD

	Cooking Time: 10 Minutes	**Servings:** 6

Ingredients	Ingredients	Directions
✓ lemon juice, 1 large lemon ✓ 1/3 cup extra-virgin olive oil ✓ 1 tsp dill weed ✓ 1 tsp garlic powder ✓ salt ✓ pepper ✓ 2 cups Pearl Couscous ✓ 2 tbsp extra virgin olive oil ✓ 2 cups grape tomatoes, halved ✓ water as needed	✓ 1/3 cup red onions, finely chopped ✓ ½ English cucumber, finely chopped ✓ 1 15-ounce can chickpeas ✓ 1 14-ounce can artichoke hearts, roughly chopped ✓ ½ cup pitted Kalamata olives ✓ 15-20 pieces fresh basil leaves, roughly torn and chopped ✓ 3 ounces fresh mozzarella	❖ Start by preparing the vinaigrette by mixing all Ingredients: in a bowl. Set aside. ❖ Heat olive oil in a medium-sized heavy pot over medium heat. ❖ Add couscous and cook until golden brown. ❖ Add 3 cups of boiling water and cook the couscous according to package instructions. ❖ Once done, drain in a colander and put it to the side. ❖ In a large mixing bowl, add the rest of the Ingredients: except the cheese and basil. ❖ Add the cooked couscous, basil, and mix everything well. ❖ Give the vinaigrette a gentle stir and whisk it into the couscous salad. Mix well. ❖ Adjust/add seasoning as desired. ❖ Add mozzarella cheese. ❖ Garnish with some basil. ❖ Enjoy!

44) EGG CUPS WITH TOMATO AND MUSHROOMS

	Cooking Time: 5 Minutes	**Servings:** 4

Ingredients	Ingredients	Directions
✓ 4 eggs ✓ 1/2 cup tomatoes, chopped ✓ 1/2 cup mushrooms, chopped ✓ 2 tbsp fresh parsley, chopped	✓ 1/4 cup half and half ✓ 1/2 cup cheddar cheese, shredded ✓ Pepper ✓ Salt	❖ In a bowl, whisk the egg with half and half, pepper, and salt. ❖ Add tomato, mushrooms, parsley, and cheese and stir well. ❖ Pour egg mixture into the four small jars and seal jars with lid. ❖ Pour 1 1/2 cups of water into the instant pot then place steamer rack in the pot. ❖ Place jars on top of the steamer rack. ❖ Seal pot with lid and cook on high for 5 minutes. ❖ Once done, release pressure using quick release. Remove lid. ❖ Serve and enjoy.

45) ITALIAN SALAD FOR BREAKFAST

	Cooking Time: 10 Minutes	**Servings:** 2

Ingredients	Ingredients	Directions
✓ 4 eggs (optional) ✓ 10 cups arugula ✓ 1/2 seedless cucumber, chopped ✓ 1 cup cooked quinoa, cooled ✓ 1 large avocado ✓ 1 cup natural almonds, chopped	✓ 1/2 cup mixed herbs like mint and dill, chopped ✓ 2 cups halved cherry tomatoes and/or heirloom tomatoes cut into wedges ✓ Extra virgin olive oil ✓ 1 lemon ✓ Sea salt, to taste ✓ Freshly ground black pepper, to taste	**Directions:** ❖ Cook the eggs by soft-boiling them - Bring a pot of water to a boil, then reduce heat to a simmer. Gently lower all the eggs into water and allow them to simmer for 6 minutes. Remove the eggs from water and run cold water on top to stop the cooking, process set aside and peel when ready to use ❖ In a large bowl, combine the arugula, tomatoes, cucumber, and quinoa ❖ Divide the salad among 2 containers, store in the fridge for 2 days ❖ To Serve: Garnish with the sliced avocado and halved egg, sprinkle herbs and almonds over top. Drizzle with olive oil, season with salt and pepper, toss to combine. Season with more salt and pepper to taste, a squeeze of lemon juice, and a drizzle of olive oil

46) SPECIAL CAULIFLOWER FRITTERS AND HUMMUS

	Cooking Time: 15 Minutes	Servings: 4

Ingredients:

- ✓ 2 (15 oz) cans chickpeas, divided
- ✓ 2 1/2 tbsp olive oil, divided, plus more for frying
- ✓ 1 cup onion, chopped, about 1/2 a small onion
- ✓ 2 tbsp garlic, minced

- ✓ 2 cups cauliflower, cut into small pieces, about 1/2 a large head
- ✓ 1/2 tsp salt
- ✓ black pepper
- ✓ Topping:
- ✓ Hummus, of choice
- ✓ Green onion, diced

Directions:

- ❖ Preheat oven to 400°F
- ❖ Rinse and drain 1 can of the chickpeas, place them on a paper towel to dry off well
- ❖ Then place the chickpeas into a large bowl, removing the loose skins that come off, and toss with 1 tbsp of olive oil, spread the chickpeas onto a large pan (being careful not to over-crowd them) and sprinkle with salt and pepper
- ❖ Bake for 20 minutes, then stir, and then bake an additional 5-10 minutes until very crispy
- ❖ Once the chickpeas are roasted, transfer them to a large food processor and process until broken down and crumble - Don't over process them and turn it into flour, as you need to have some texture. Place the mixture into a small bowl, set aside
- ❖ In a large pan over medium-high heat, add the remaining 1 1/2 tbsp of olive oil
- ❖ Once heated, add in the onion and garlic, cook until lightly golden brown, about 2 minutes. Then add in the chopped cauliflower, cook for an additional 2 minutes, until the cauliflower is golden
- ❖ Turn the heat down to low and cover the pan, cook until the cauliflower is fork tender and the onions are golden brown and caramelized, stirring often, about 3-5 minutes
- ❖ Transfer the cauliflower mixture to the food processor, drain and rinse the remaining can of chickpeas and add them into the food processor, along with the salt and a pinch of pepper. Blend until smooth, and the mixture starts to ball, stop to scrape down the sides as needed
- ❖ Transfer the cauliflower mixture into a large bowl and add in 1/2 cup of the roasted chickpea crumbs (you won't use all of the crumbs, but it is easier to break them down when you have a larger amount.), stir until well combined
- ❖ In a large bowl over medium heat, add in enough oil to lightly cover the bottom of a large pan
- ❖ Working in batches, cook the patties until golden brown, about 2-3 minutes, flip and cook again
- ❖ Distribute among the container, placing parchment paper in between the fritters. Store in the fridge for 2-3 days
- ❖ To Serve: Heat through in the oven at 350F for 5-8 minutes. Top with hummus, green onion and enjoy!
- ❖ Recipe Notes: Don't add too much oil while frying the fritter or they will end up soggy. Use only enough to cover the pan. Use a fork while frying and resist the urge to flip them every minute to see if they are golden

Nutrition: Calories:333;Total Carbohydrates: 45g;Total Fat: 13g;Protein: 14g

47) ITALIAN BREAKFAST SAUSAGE AND NEW POTATOES WITH VEGETABLES

		Cooking Time: 30 Minutes	Servings: 4

✓ 1 lbs sweet Italian sausage links, sliced on the bias (diagonal) ✓ 2 cups baby potatoes, halved ✓ 2 cups broccoli florets ✓ 1 cup onions cut to 1-inch chunks ✓ 2 cups small mushrooms -half or quarter the large ones for uniform size	✓ 1 cup baby carrots ✓ 2 tbsp olive oil ✓ 1/2 tsp garlic powder ✓ 1/2 tsp Italian seasoning ✓ 1 tsp salt ✓ 1/2 tsp pepper	❖ Preheat the oven to 400 degrees F ❖ In a large bowl, add the baby potatoes, broccoli florets, onions, small mushrooms, and baby carrots ❖ Add in the olive oil, salt, pepper, garlic powder and Italian seasoning and toss to evenly coat ❖ Spread the vegetables onto a sheet pan in one even layer ❖ Arrange the sausage slices on the pan over the vegetables ❖ Bake for 30 minutes – make sure to sake halfway through to prevent sticking ❖ Allow to cool ❖ Distribute the Italian sausages and vegetables among the containers and store in the fridge for 2-3 days ❖ To Serve: Reheat in the microwave for 1-2 minutes, or until heated through and enjoy! ❖ Recipe Notes: If you would like crispier potatoes, place them on the pan and bake for 15 minutes before adding the other ingredients to the pan.

48) GREEK QUINOA BREAKFAST BOWL

		Cooking Time: 20 Minutes	Servings: 6

✓ 12 eggs ✓ ¼ cup plain Greek yogurt ✓ 1 tsp onion powder ✓ 1 tsp granulated garlic ✓ ½ tsp salt ✓ ½ tsp pepper	✓ 1 tsp olive oil ✓ 1 (5 oz) bag baby spinach ✓ 1 pint cherry tomatoes, halved ✓ 1 cup feta cheese ✓ 2 cups cooked quinoa	❖ In a large bowl whisk together eggs, Greek yogurt, onion powder, granulated garlic, salt, and pepper, set aside ❖ In a large skillet, heat olive oil and add spinach, cook the spinach until it is slightly wilted, about 3-4 minutes. Add in cherry tomatoes, cook until tomatoes are softened, 4 minutes. Stir in egg mixture and cook until the eggs are set, about 7-9 minutes, stir in the eggs as they cook to scramble ❖ Once the eggs have set stir in the feta and quinoa, cook until heated through. Distribute evenly among the containers, store for 2-3 days ❖ To serve: Reheat in the microwave for 30 seconds to 1 minute or heated through

49) EGG, HAM AND CHEESE SANDWICHES IN THE FREEZER

		Cooking Time: 20 Minutes	Servings: 6

✓ Cooking spray or oil to grease the baking dish ✓ 7 large eggs ✓ ½ cup low-fat (2%) milk ✓ ½ tsp garlic powder ✓ ½ tsp onion powder	✓ 1 tbsp Dijon mustard ✓ ½ tsp honey ✓ 6 whole-wheat English muffins ✓ 6 slices thinly sliced prosciutto ✓ 6 slices Swiss cheese	❖ Preheat the oven to 375°F. Lightly oil or spray an 8-by--inch glass or ceramic baking dish with cooking spray. ❖ In a large bowl, whisk together the eggs, milk, garlic powder, and onion powder. Pour the mixture into the baking dish and bake for minutes, until the eggs are set and no longer jiggling. Cool. ❖ While the eggs are baking, mix the mustard and honey in a small bowl. Lay out the English muffin halves to start assembly. ❖ When the eggs are cool, use a biscuit cutter or drinking glass about the same size as the English muffin diameter to cut 6 egg circles. Divide the leftover egg scraps evenly to be added to each sandwich. ❖ Spread ½ tsp of honey mustard on each of the bottom English muffin halves. Top each with 1 slice of prosciutto, 1 egg circle and scraps, 1 slice of cheese, and the top half of the muffin. ❖ Wrap each sandwich tightly in foil. ❖

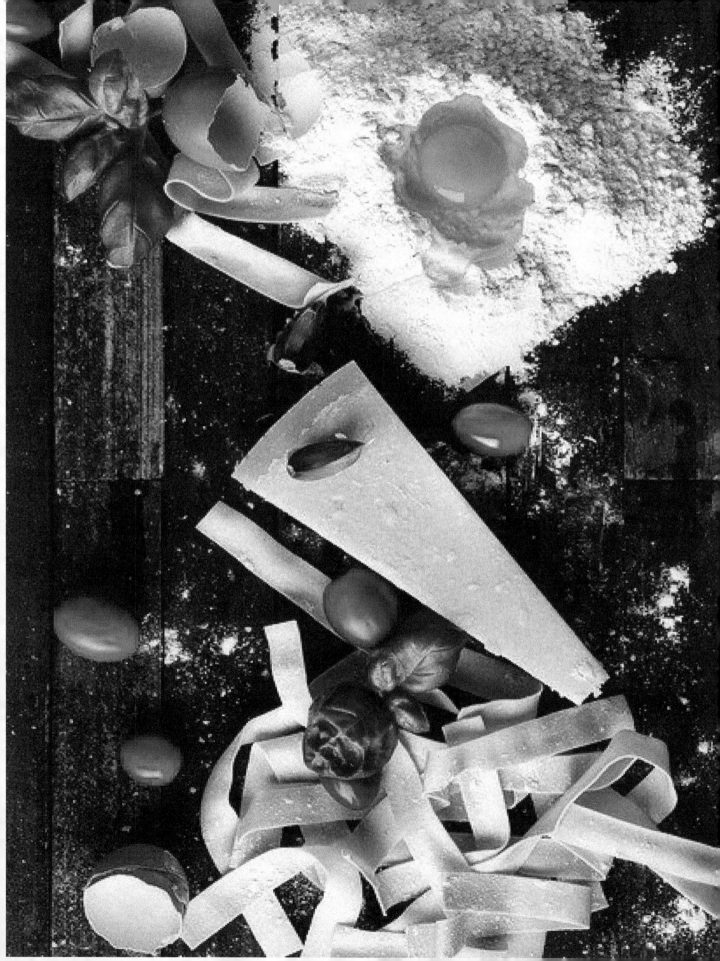

50) HEALTHY SALAD ZUCCHINI CABBAGE TOMATO

	Cooking Time: 20 Minutes	Servings: 4

Ingredients:

- ✓ 1 lb kale, chopped
- ✓ 2 tbsp fresh parsley, chopped
- ✓ 1 tbsp vinegar
- ✓ 1/2 cup can tomato, crushed
- ✓ 1 tsp paprika
- ✓ 1 cup zucchini, cut into cubes
- ✓ 1 cup grape tomatoes, halved
- ✓ 2 tbsp olive oil
- ✓ 1 onion, chopped
- ✓ 1 leek, sliced
- ✓ Pepper
- ✓ Salt

Directions:

- ❖ Add oil into the inner pot of instant pot and set the pot on sauté mode.
- ❖ Add leek and onion and sauté for 5 minutes.
- ❖ Add kale and remaining ingredients and stir well.
- ❖ Seal pot with lid and cook on high for 15 minutes.
- ❖ Once done, allow to release pressure naturally for 10 minutes then release remaining using quick release. Remove lid.
- ❖ Stir and serve.

Nutrition: Calories: 162;Fat: 3 g;Carbohydrates: 22.2 g;Sugar: 4.8 g;Protein: 5.2 g;Cholesterol: 0 mg

51) Bacon Brie omelette with radish salad

	Cooking Time: 10 Minutes	Servings: 6

Ingredients:

- ✓ 200 g smoked lardons
- ✓ 3 tsp olive oil, divided
- ✓ 7 ounces smoked bacon
- ✓ 6 lightly beaten eggs
- ✓ small bunch chives, snipped up
- ✓ 3½ ounces sliced brie
- ✓ 1 tsp red wine vinegar
- ✓ 1 tsp Dijon mustard
- ✓ 1 cucumber, deseeded, halved, and sliced up diagonally
- ✓ 7 ounces radish, quartered

Directions:

- ❖ Heat up the grill.
- ❖ Add 1 tsp of oil to a small pan and heat on the grill.
- ❖ Add lardons and fry them until nice and crisp.
- ❖ Drain the lardon on kitchen paper.
- ❖ Heat the remaining 2 tsp of oil in a non-sticking pan on the grill.
- ❖ Add lardons, eggs, chives, and ground pepper, and cook over low heat until semi-set.
- ❖ Carefully lay the Brie on top, and grill until it has set and is golden in color.
- ❖ Remove from pan and cut into wedges.
- ❖ Make the salad by mixing olive oil, mustard, vinegar, and seasoning in a bowl.
- ❖ Add cucumber and radish and mix well.
- ❖ Serve the salad alongside the Omelette wedges in containers.
- ❖ Enjoy!

52) OATMEAL WITH CRANBERRIES

	Cooking Time: 6 Minutes	**Servings:** 2

Ingredients:		Directions:
✓ 1/2 cup steel-cut oats ✓ 1 cup unsweetened almond milk ✓ 1 1/2 tbsp maple syrup ✓ 1/4 tsp cinnamon	✓ 1/4 tsp vanilla ✓ 1/4 cup dried cranberries ✓ 1 cup of water ✓ 1 tsp lemon zest, grated ✓ 1/4 cup orange juice	❖ Add all ingredients into the heat-safe dish and stir well. ❖ Pour 1 cup of water into the instant pot then place the trivet in the pot. ❖ Place dish on top of the trivet. ❖ Seal pot with lid and cook on high for 6 minutes. ❖ Once done, allow to release pressure naturally for 10 minutes then release remaining using quick release. Remove lid. ❖ Serve and enjoy.

Nutrition: Calories: 161;Fat: 3.2 g;Carbohydrates: 29.9 g;Sugar: 12.4 g;Protein: 3.4 g;Cholesterol: 0 mg

53) FIGS TOAST WITH RICOTTA CHEESE

	Cooking Time: 15 Minutes	**Servings:** 1

Ingredients:		Directions:
✓ 2 slices whole-wheat toast ✓ 1 tsp honey ✓ ¼ cup ricotta (partly skimmed)	✓ 1 dash cinnamon ✓ 2 figs (sliced) ✓ 1 tsp sesame seeds	❖ Start by mixing ricotta with honey and dash of cinnamon. ❖ Then, spread this mixture on the toast. ❖ Now, top with fig and sesame seeds. ❖ Serve.

54) QUICK SPINACH, FETA WITH EGG BREAKFAST QUESADILLAS

	Cooking Time: 15 Minutes	**Servings:** 5

Ingredients:		Directions:
✓ 8 eggs (optional) ✓ 2 tsp olive oil ✓ 1 red bell pepper ✓ 1/2 red onion ✓ 1/4 cup milk	✓ 4 handfuls of spinach leaves ✓ 1 1/2 cup mozzarella cheese ✓ 5 sun-dried tomato tortillas ✓ 1/2 cup feta ✓ 1/4 tsp salt ✓ 1/4 tsp pepper ✓ Spray oil	❖ In a large non-stick pan over medium heat, add the olive oil ❖ Once heated, add the bell pepper and onion, cook for 4-5 minutes until soft ❖ In the meantime, whisk together the eggs, milk, salt and pepper in a bowl ❖ Add in the egg/milk mixture into the pan with peppers and onions, stirring frequently, until eggs are almost cooked through ❖ Add in the spinach and feta, fold into the eggs, stirring until spinach is wilted and eggs are cooked through ❖ Remove the eggs from heat and plate ❖ Spray a separate large non-stick pan with spray oil, and place over medium heat ❖ Add the tortilla, on one half of the tortilla, spread about ½ cup of the egg mixture ❖ Top the eggs with around ⅓ cup of shredded mozzarella cheese ❖ Fold the second half of the tortilla over, then cook for 2 minutes, or until golden brown ❖ Flip and cook for another minute until golden brown ❖ Allow the quesadilla to cool completely, divide among the container, store for 2 days or wrap in plastic wrap and foil, and freeze for up to 2 months ❖ To Serve: Reheat in oven at 375 for 3-5 minutes or until heated through

Nutrition: (1/2 quesadilla): Calories:213;Total Fat: 11g;Total Carbs: 15g;Protein: 15g

55) BREAKFAST COBBLER

Cooking Time: 12 Minutes   **Servings:** 4

Ingredients:

- ✓ 2 lbs apples, cut into chunks
- ✓ 1 1/2 cups water
- ✓ 1/4 tsp nutmeg
- ✓ 1 1/2 tsp cinnamon
- ✓ 1/2 cup dry buckwheat
- ✓ 1/2 cup dates, chopped
- ✓ Pinch of ground ginger

Directions:

- ❖ Spray instant pot from inside with cooking spray.
- ❖ Add all ingredients into the instant pot and stir well.
- ❖ Seal pot with a lid and select manual and set timer for 12 minutes.
- ❖ Once done, release pressure using quick release. Remove lid.
- ❖ Stir and serve.

Nutrition: Calories: 195;Fat: 0.9 g;Carbohydrates: 48.3 g;Sugar: 25.8 g;Protein: 3.3 g;Cholesterol: 0 mg

57) EGG QUINOA AND KALE BOWL

Cooking Time: 5 Minutes   **Servings:** 2

Ingredients:

- ✓ 1-ounce pancetta, chopped
- ✓ 1 bunch kale, sliced
- ✓ ½ cup cherry tomatoes, halved
- ✓ 1 tsp red wine vinegar
- ✓ 1 cup cooked quinoa
- ✓ 1 tsp olive oil
- ✓ 2 eggs
- ✓ 1/3 cup avocado, sliced
- ✓ sea salt or plain salt
- ✓ fresh black pepper

Directions:

- ❖ Start by heating pancetta in a skillet until golden brown. Add in kale and further cook for 2 minutes.
- ❖ Then, stir in tomatoes, vinegar, and salt and remove from heat.
- ❖ Now, divide this mixture into 2 bowls, add avocado to both, and then set aside.
- ❖ Finally, cook both the eggs and top each bowl with an egg.
- ❖ Serve hot with toppings of your choice.

58) GREEK STRAWBERRY COLD YOGURT

Cooking Time: 2-4 Hours   **Servings:** 5

Ingredients:

- ✓ 3 cups plain Greek low-fat yogurt
- ✓ 1 cup sugar
- ✓ ¼ cup lemon juice, freshly squeezed
- ✓ 2 tsp vanilla
- ✓ 1/8 tsp salt
- ✓ 1 cup strawberries, sliced

Directions:

- ❖ In a medium-sized bowl, add yogurt, lemon juice, sugar, vanilla, and salt.
- ❖ Whisk the whole mixture well.
- ❖ Freeze the yogurt mix in a 2-quart ice cream maker according to the given instructions.
- ❖ During the final minute, add the sliced strawberries.
- ❖ Transfer the yogurt to an airtight container.
- ❖ Place in the freezer for 2-4 hours.
- ❖ Remove from the freezer and allow it to stand for 5-15 minutes.
- ❖ Serve and enjoy!

Nutrition: Calories: 251, Total Fat: 0.5 g, Saturated Fat: 0.1 g, Cholesterol: 3 mg, Sodium: 130 mg, Total Carbohydrate: 48.7 g, Dietary Fiber: 0.6 g, Total Sugars: 47.3 g, Protein: 14.7 g, Vitamin D: 1 mcg, Calcium: 426 mg, Iron: 0 mg, Potassium: 62 mg

59) SPECIAL PEACH ALMOND OATMEAL

	Cooking Time: 10 Minutes	Servings: 2

✓ 1 cup unsweetened almond milk ✓ 2 cups of water	✓ 1 cup oats ✓ 2 peaches, diced ✓ Pinch of salt	❖ Spray instant pot from inside with cooking spray. ❖ Add all ingredients into the instant pot and stir well. ❖ Seal pot with a lid and select manual and set timer for 10 minutes. ❖ Once done, allow to release pressure naturally for 10 minutes then release remaining using quick release. Remove lid. Stir and serve.

60) EVERYDAY BANANA PEANUT BUTTER PUDDING

	Cooking Time: 25 Minutes	Servings: 1

✓ 2 bananas, halved ✓ ¼ cup smooth peanut butter	✓ Coconut for garnish, shredded	❖ Start by blending bananas and peanut butter in a blender and mix until smooth or desired texture obtained. ❖ Pour into a bowl and garnish with coconut if desired. Enjoy.

61) SPECIAL COCONUT BANANA MIX

	Cooking Time: 4 Minutes	Servings: 4

✓ 1 cup coconut milk ✓ 1 banana ✓ 1 cup dried coconut ✓ 2 tbsp ground flax seed	✓ 3 tbsp chopped raisins ✓ ⅛ tsp nutmeg ✓ ⅛ tsp cinnamon ✓ Salt to taste	❖ Set a large skillet on the stove and set it to low heat. ❖ Chop up the banana. ❖ Pour the coconut milk, nutmeg, and cinnamon into the skillet. ❖ Pour in the ground flaxseed while stirring continuously. ❖ Add the dried coconut and banana. Mix the ingredients until combined well. ❖ Allow the mixture to simmer for 2 to 3 minutes while stirring occasionally. ❖ Set four airtight containers on the counter. ❖ Remove the pan from heat and sprinkle enough salt for your taste buds. ❖ Divide the mixture into the containers and place them into the fridge overnight. They can remain in the fridge for up to 3 days. ❖ Before you set this tasty mixture in the microwave to heat up, you need to let it thaw on the counter for a bit.

62) RASPBERRY AND LEMON MUFFINS WITH OLIVE OIL

	Cooking Time: 20 Minutes	Servings: 12

✓ Cooking spray to grease baking liners ✓ 1 cup all-purpose flour ✓ 1 cup whole-wheat flour ✓ ½ cup tightly packed light brown sugar ✓ ½ tsp baking soda ✓ ½ tsp aluminum-free baking powder	✓ ⅛ tsp kosher salt ✓ 1¼ cups buttermilk ✓ 1 large egg ✓ ¼ cup extra-virgin olive oil ✓ 1 tbsp freshly squeezed lemon juice ✓ Zest of 2 lemons ✓ 1¼ cups frozen raspberries (do not thaw)	❖ Preheat the oven to 400°F and line a muffin tin with baking liners. Spray the liners lightly with cooking spray. ❖ In a large mixing bowl, whisk together the all-purpose flour, whole-wheat flour, brown sugar, baking soda, baking powder, and salt. ❖ In a medium bowl, whisk together the buttermilk, egg, oil, lemon juice, and lemon zest. ❖ Pour the wet ingredients into the dry ingredients and stir just until blended. Do not overmix. ❖ Fold in the frozen raspberries. ❖ Scoop about ¼ cup of batter into each muffin liner and bake for 20 minutes, or until the tops look browned and a paring knife comes out clean when inserted. Remove the muffins from the tin to cool. ❖ STORAGE: Store covered containers at room temperature for up to 4 days. To freeze muffins for up to 3 months, wrap them in foil and place in an airtight resealable bag.

63) EASY COUSCOUS PEARL SALAD

		Cooking Time: 10 Minutes		Servings: 6

Ingredients	Ingredients	Directions
✓ lemon juice, 1 large lemon ✓ 1/3 cup extra-virgin olive oil ✓ 1 tsp dill weed ✓ 1 tsp garlic powder ✓ salt ✓ pepper ✓ 2 cups Pearl Couscous ✓ 2 tbsp extra virgin olive oil ✓ 2 cups grape tomatoes, halved ✓ water as needed	✓ 1/3 cup red onions, finely chopped ✓ ½ English cucumber, finely chopped ✓ 1 15-ounce can chickpeas ✓ 1 14-ounce can artichoke hearts, roughly chopped ✓ ½ cup pitted Kalamata olives ✓ 15-20 pieces fresh basil leaves, roughly torn and chopped ✓ 3 ounces fresh mozzarella	❖ Start by preparing the vinaigrette by mixing all Ingredients: in a bowl. Set aside. ❖ Heat olive oil in a medium-sized heavy pot over medium heat. ❖ Add couscous and cook until golden brown. ❖ Add 3 cups of boiling water and cook the couscous according to package instructions. ❖ Once done, drain in a colander and put it to the side. ❖ In a large mixing bowl, add the rest of the Ingredients: except the cheese and basil. ❖ Add the cooked couscous, basil, and mix everything well. ❖ Give the vinaigrette a gentle stir and whisk it into the couscous salad. Mix well. ❖ Adjust/add seasoning as desired. ❖ Add mozzarella cheese. ❖ Garnish with some basil. ❖ Enjoy!

64) EGG CUPS WITH TOMATO AND MUSHROOMS

		Cooking Time: 5 Minutes		Servings: 4

Ingredients	Ingredients	Directions
✓ 4 eggs ✓ 1/2 cup tomatoes, chopped ✓ 1/2 cup mushrooms, chopped ✓ 2 tbsp fresh parsley, chopped	✓ 1/4 cup half and half ✓ 1/2 cup cheddar cheese, shredded ✓ Pepper ✓ Salt	❖ In a bowl, whisk the egg with half and half, pepper, and salt. ❖ Add tomato, mushrooms, parsley, and cheese and stir well. ❖ Pour egg mixture into the four small jars and seal jars with lid. ❖ Pour 1 1/2 cups of water into the instant pot then place steamer rack in the pot. ❖ Place jars on top of the steamer rack. ❖ Seal pot with lid and cook on high for 5 minutes. ❖ Once done, release pressure using quick release. Remove lid. ❖ Serve and enjoy.

65) ITALIAN SALAD FOR BREAKFAST

		Cooking Time: 10 Minutes		Servings: 2

Ingredients	Ingredients	Directions
✓ 4 eggs (optional) ✓ 10 cups arugula ✓ 1/2 seedless cucumber, chopped ✓ 1 cup cooked quinoa, cooled ✓ 1 large avocado ✓ 1 cup natural almonds, chopped	✓ 1/2 cup mixed herbs like mint and dill, chopped ✓ 2 cups halved cherry tomatoes and/or heirloom tomatoes cut into wedges ✓ Extra virgin olive oil ✓ 1 lemon ✓ Sea salt, to taste ✓ Freshly ground black pepper, to taste	**Directions:** ❖ Cook the eggs by soft-boiling them - Bring a pot of water to a boil, then reduce heat to a simmer. Gently lower all the eggs into water and allow them to simmer for 6 minutes. Remove the eggs from water and run cold water on top to stop the cooking, process set aside and peel when ready to use ❖ In a large bowl, combine the arugula, tomatoes, cucumber, and quinoa ❖ Divide the salad among 2 containers, store in the fridge for 2 days ❖ To Serve: Garnish with the sliced avocado and halved egg, sprinkle herbs and almonds over top. Drizzle with olive oil, season with salt and pepper, toss to combine. Season with more salt and pepper to taste, a squeeze of lemon juice, and a drizzle of olive oil

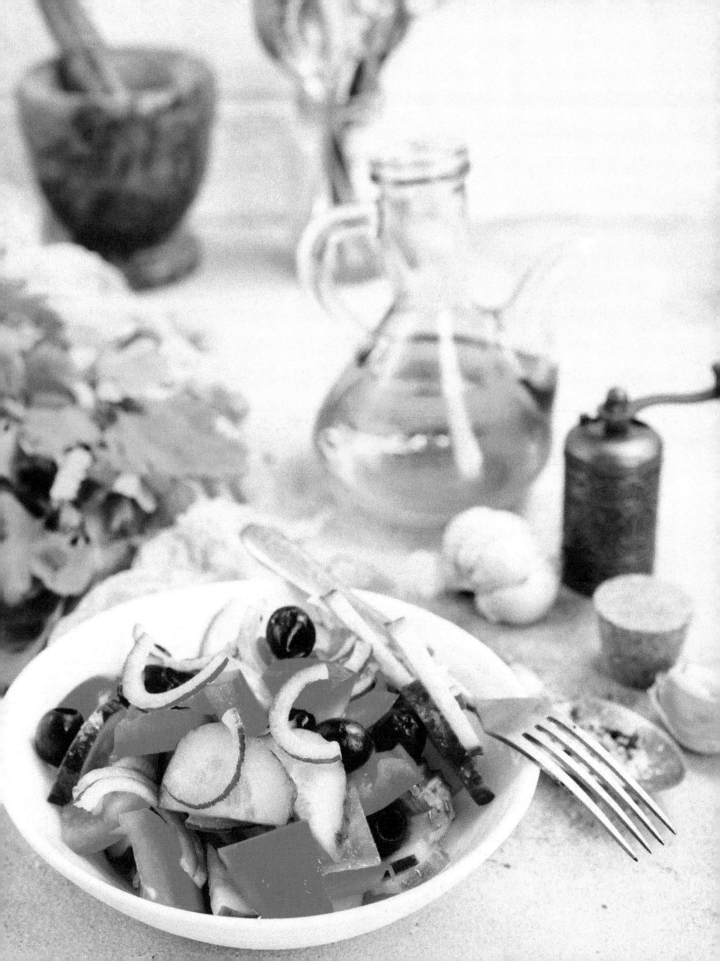

Chapter 2. LUNCH

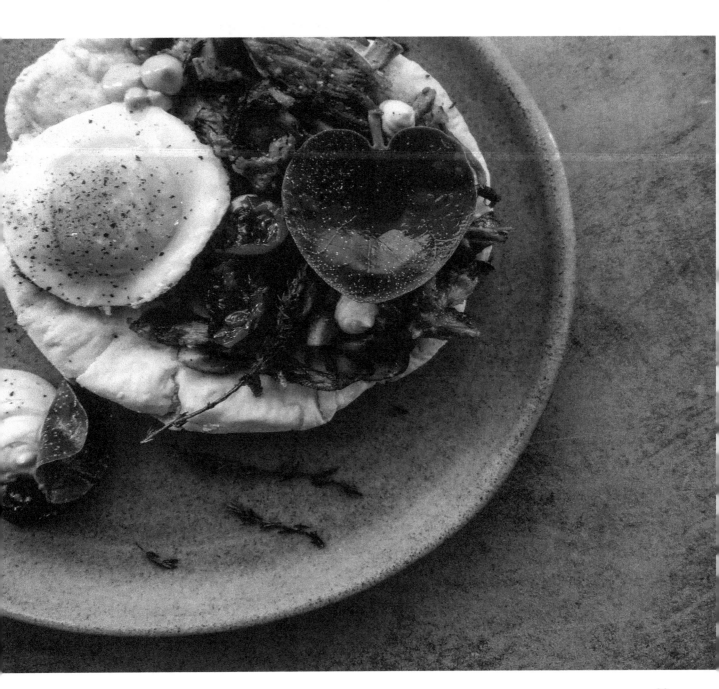

66) SPECIAL FRUIT SALAD WITH MINT AND ORANGE BLOSSOM WATER

	Cooking Time: 10 Minutes	Servings: 5

Ingredients:

- ✓ 3 cups cantaloupe, cut into 1-inch cubes
- ✓ 2 cups hulled and halved strawberries
- ✓ ½ tsp orange blossom water
- ✓ 2 tbsp chopped fresh mint

Directions:

- ❖ In a large bowl, toss all the ingredients together.
- ❖ Place 1 cup of fruit salad in each of 5 containers.
- ❖ STORAGE: Store covered containers in the refrigerator for up to 5 days.

Nutrition: Total calories: 52; Total fat: 1g; Saturated fat: <1g; Sodium: 10mg; Carbohydrates: 12g; Fiber: 2g; Protein: 1g

67) ROASTED BROCCOLI WITH RED ONIONS AND POMEGRANATE SEEDS

	Cooking Time: 20 Minutes	Servings: 5

Ingredients:

- ✓ 1 (12-ounce) package broccoli florets (about 6 cups)
- ✓ 1 small red onion, thinly sliced
- ✓ 2 tbsp olive oil
- ✓ ¼ tsp kosher salt
- ✓ 1 (5.3-ounce) container pomegranate seeds (1 cup)

Directions:

- ❖ Preheat the oven to 425°F and line 2 sheet pans with silicone baking mats or parchment paper.
- ❖ Place the broccoli and onion on the sheet pans and toss with the oil and salt. Place the pans in the oven and roast for minutes.
- ❖ After removing the pans from the oven, cool the veggies, then toss with the pomegranate seeds.
- ❖ Place 1 cup of veggies in each of 5 containers.
- ❖ STORAGE: Store covered containers in the refrigerator for up to days.

Nutrition: Total calories: 118; Total fat: ; Saturated fat: 1g; Sodium: 142mg; Carbohydrates: 12g; Fiber: 4g; Protein: 2g

68) DELICIOUS CHERMOULA SAUCE

	Cooking Time: 10 Minutes	Servings: 1 Cup

Ingredients:

- ✓ 1 cup packed parsley leaves
- ✓ 1 cup cilantro leaves
- ✓ ½ cup mint leaves
- ✓ 1 tsp chopped garlic
- ✓ ½ tsp ground cumin
- ✓ ½ tsp ground coriander
- ✓ ½ tsp smoked paprika
- ✓ ⅛ tsp cayenne pepper
- ✓ ⅛ tsp kosher salt
- ✓ 3 tbsp freshly squeezed lemon juice
- ✓ 3 tbsp water
- ✓ ½ cup extra-virgin olive oil

Directions:

- ❖ Place all the ingredients in a blender or food processor and blend until smooth.
- ❖ Pour the chermoula into a container and refrigerate.
- ❖ STORAGE: Store the covered container in the refrigerator for up to 5 days.

Nutrition: (¼ cup): Total calories: 257; Total fat: 27g; Saturated fat: ; Sodium: 96mg; Carbohydrates: 4g; Fiber: 2g; Protein: 1g

69) DEVILED EGG PESTO WITH SUN-DRIED TOMATOES

	Cooking Time: 15 Minutes	Servings: 5

Ingredients:

- ✓ 5 large eggs
- ✓ 3 tbsp prepared pesto
- ✓ ¼ tsp white vinegar
- ✓ 2 tbsp low-fat (2%) plain Greek yogurt
- ✓ 5 tsp sliced sun-dried tomatoes

❖ Place the eggs in a saucepan and cover with water. Bring the water to a boil. As soon as the water starts to boil, place a lid on the pan and turn the heat off. Set a timer for minutes.

❖ When the timer goes off, drain the hot water and run cold water over the eggs to cool.

❖ Peel the eggs, slice in half vertically, and scoop out the yolks. Place the yolks in a medium mixing bowl and add the pesto, vinegar, and yogurt. Mix well, until creamy.

❖ Scoop about 1 tbsp of the pesto-yolk mixture into each egg half. Top each with ½ tsp of sun-dried tomatoes.

❖ Place 2 stuffed egg halves in each of separate containers.

❖ STORAGE: Store covered containers in the refrigerator for up to 5 days.

70) WHITE BEAN WITH MUSHROOM DIP

	Cooking Time: 8 Minutes	Servings: 3 Cups

Ingredients:

- ✓ 2 tsp olive oil, plus 2 tbsp
- ✓ 8 ounces button or cremini mushrooms, sliced
- ✓ 1 tsp chopped garlic
- ✓ 1 tbsp fresh thyme leaves
- ✓ 2 (15.5-ounce) cans cannellini beans, drained and rinsed
- ✓ 2 tbsp plus 1 tsp freshly squeezed lemon juice
- ✓ ½ tsp kosher salt

❖ Heat 2 tsp of oil in a -inch skillet over medium-high heat. Once the oil is shimmering, add the mushrooms and sauté for 6 minutes. Add the garlic and thyme and continue cooking for 2 minutes.

❖ While the mushrooms are cooking, place the beans and lemon juice, the remaining tbsp of oil, and the salt in the bowl of a food processor. Add the mushrooms as soon as they are done cooking and blend everything until smooth. Scrape down the sides of the bowl if necessary and continue to process until smooth.

❖ Taste and adjust the seasoning with lemon juice or salt if needed.

❖ Scoop the dip into a container and refrigerate.

❖ STORAGE: Store the covered container in the refrigerator for up to days. Dip can be frozen for up to 3 months.

71) SPICY SAUTÉED CABBAGE IN NORTH AFRICAN STYLE

	Cooking Time: 10 Minutes	Servings: 4

Ingredients:

- ✓ 2 tsp olive oil
- ✓ 1 small head green cabbage (about 1½ to 2 pounds), cored and thinly sliced
- ✓ 1 tsp ground coriander
- ✓ 1 tsp garlic powder
- ✓ ½ tsp caraway seeds
- ✓ ½ tsp ground cumin
- ✓ ¼ tsp kosher salt
- ✓ Pinch red chili flakes (optional—if you don't like heat, omit it)
- ✓ 1 tsp freshly squeezed lemon juice

Directions:

❖ Heat the oil in a -inch skillet over medium-high heat. Once the oil is hot, add the cabbage and cook down for 3 minutes. Add the coriander, garlic powder, caraway seeds, cumin, salt, and chili flakes (if using) and stir to combine. Continue cooking the cabbage for about 7 more minutes.

❖ Stir in the lemon juice and cool.

❖ Place 1 heaping cup of cabbage in each of 4 containers.

❖ STORAGE: Store covered containers in the refrigerator for up to 5 days.

72) ROAST VEGETABLE QUINOA BOWL

	Cooking Time: 20 Minutes	**Servings: 2**

✓ Quinoa: ✓ ¾ cup quinoa, rinsed ✓ 1 ½ cups ✓ vegetable broth ✓ Chili-Lime Kale ✓ 1/2 tsp chili powder ✓ pinch salt ✓ pinch pepper ✓ 2 cups packed kale, de-stemmed and chopped ✓ 1 tsp olive, coconut or canola oil ✓ Juice of 1/4 lime ✓ Garlic Roasted Broccoli: ✓ 2 cups broccoli, ✓ 2 tsp olive or canola oil ✓ 2 cloves garlic, minced ✓ Pinch of salt	✓ Black pepper ✓ Curry Roasted Sweet Potatoes: ✓ 1 small sweet potato ✓ 1 tsp olive or canola oil ✓ 1 tsp curry powder ✓ 1 tsp sriracha ✓ Pinch salt ✓ Spicy Roasted Chickpeas: ✓ 1 ½ cups (cooked) chickpeas ✓ 1 tsp olive or canola oil ✓ 2 tsp sriracha ✓ 2 tsp soy sauce ✓ Optional: ✓ Lime ✓ Avocado ✓ Hummus ✓ Red pepper flakes ✓ Guacamole	❖ Preheat the oven to 400-degree F ❖ Line a large baking sheet with parchment paper ❖ Prepare the vegetables by chopping the broccoli into medium sized florets, de-stemming and chopping the kale, scrubbing and slicing the sweet potato into ¼" wide rounds ❖ Take the broccoli florets and massage with oil, garlic, salt and pepper - making sure to work the ingredients into the tops of each florets - Place the florets in a row down in the center third of a large baking sheet ❖ Using the same bowl, the broccoli in, mix together the chickpeas, oil, sriracha and soy sauce, then spread them out in a row next to the broccoli ❖ In the same bowl combine the oil, curry powder, salt, and sriracha, add the sliced sweet potato and toss to coat, then lay the rounds on the remaining third of the baking tray ❖ Bake for 10 minutes, flip the sweet potatoes and broccoli, and redistribute the chickpeas to cook evenly Bake for another 8-12 minutes ❖ For the Quinoa: Prepare the quinoa by rinsing and draining it. Add the rinsed quinoa and vegetable broth to a small saucepan and bring to a boil over high heat. Turn the heat down to medium-low, cover and allow to simmer for about 15 minutes. Once cooked, fluff with a fork and set aside ❖ In the meantime, place a large skillet with 1 tsp oil, add in the kale and cook for about 5 minutes, or until nearly tender ❖ Add in the salt, chili powder, and lime juice, toss to coat and cook for another 2-3 minutes ❖ Allow all the ingredient to cool ❖ Distribute among the containers – Add ½ to 1 cup of quinoa into each bowl, top with ½ of the broccoli, ½ kale, ½ the chickpeas and ½ sweet potatoes ❖ To Serve: Reheat in the microwave for 1-2 minutes or until heated through. Enjoy

Nutrition: Calories:611;Carbs: 93g;Total Fat: 17g;Protein: 24g

73) ITALIAN-STYLE SALMON

	Cooking Time: 15 Minutes	**Servings: 4**

✓ ½ cup of olive oil ✓ ¼ cup balsamic vinegar ✓ 4 garlic cloves, pressed ✓ 4 pieces salmon fillets	✓ 1 tbsp fresh cilantro, chopped ✓ 1 tbsp fresh basil, chopped ✓ 1½ tsp garlic salt	❖ Combine olive oil and balsamic vinegar. ❖ Add salmon fillets to a shallow baking dish. ❖ Rub the garlic onto the fillets. ❖ Pour vinegar and oil all over, making sure to turn them once to coat them. ❖ Season with cilantro, garlic salt, and basil. ❖ Set aside and allow to marinate for about 10 minutes. ❖ Preheat the broiler to your oven. ❖ Place the baking dish with the salmon about 6 inches from the heat source. ❖ Broil for 15 minutes until both sides are evenly browned and can be flaked with a fork. ❖ Make sure to keep brushing with sauce from the pan. ❖ Enjoy!

Nutrition: Calories: 459, Total Fat: 36.2 g, Saturated Fat: 5.2 g, Cholesterol: 78 mg, Sodium: 80 mg, Total Carbohydrate: 1.2 g, Dietary Fiber: 0.1 g, Total Sugars: 0.1 g, Protein: 34.8 g, Vitamin D: 0 mcg, Calcium: 71 mg, Iron: 1 mg, Potassium: 710 mg

74) HEARTTHROB ITALIAN-STYLE TILAPIA

		Cooking Time: 15 Minutes		Servings: 4

Ingredients	Ingredients	Directions
✓ 3 tbsp sun-dried tomatoes, packed in oil, drained and chopped ✓ 1 tbsp capers, drained ✓ 2 tilapia fillets	✓ 1 tbsp oil from sun-dried tomatoes ✓ 1 tbsp lemon juice ✓ 2 tbsp kalamata olives, chopped and pitted	❖ Pre-heat your oven to 372-degree Fahrenheit ❖ Take a small sized bowl and add sun-dried tomatoes, olives, capers and stir well ❖ Keep the mixture on the side ❖ Take a baking sheet and transfer the tilapia fillets and arrange them side by side. Drizzle olive oil all over them. Drizzle lemon juice ❖ Bake in your oven for 10-15 minutes ❖ After 10 minutes, check the fish for a "Flaky" texture ❖ Once cooked properly, top the fish with tomato mix and serve! ❖ Meal Prep/Storage Options: Store in airtight containers in your fridge for 1-3 days.

Nutrition: Calories: 183;Fat: 8g;Carbohydrates: 18g;Protein:183g

75) GARLIC WITH CAJUN SHRIMP BOWL AND NOODLES

		Cooking Time: 15 Minutes		Servings: 2

Ingredients	Ingredients	Directions
✓ 1 sliced onion ✓ 1 tbsp almond butter, but you can use regular butter as well ✓ 1 tsp onion powder ✓ ½ tsp salt ✓ 1 sliced red pepper	✓ 3 cloves of minced garlic ✓ 1 tsp paprika ✓ 20 jumbo shrimp, deveined and shells removed ✓ 3 tbsp of ghee ✓ 2 zucchini, 3 if they are smaller in size, cut into noodles ✓ Red pepper flakes and cayenne pepper, as desired	❖ In a small bowl, mix the pepper flakes, paprika, onion powder, salt, and cayenne pepper. ❖ Toss the shrimp into the cajun mixture and coat the seafood thoroughly. ❖ Add the ghee to a medium or large skillet and place on medium-low heat. ❖ Once the ghee is melted, add the garlic and saute for minutes. ❖ Carefully add the shrimp into the skillet and cook until they are opaque. Set the pan aside. ❖ In a new pan, add the butter and allow it to melt. ❖ Combine the zucchini noodles and cook on medium-low heat for 3 to 4 minutes. ❖ Turn off the heat and place the zucchini noodles on serving dishes. Add the shrimp to the top and enjoy.

Nutrition: calories: 712, fats: 30 grams, carbohydrates: 20.1 grams, protein: grams.

76) EASY MARINATED CHICKEN WITH GARLIC

		Cooking Time: 15 Minutes		Servings: 3

Ingredients	Ingredients	Directions
✓ 1 ½ lbs. boneless skinless chicken breasts, ✓ 1/4 cup olive oil ✓ 1/4 cup lemon juice ✓ 3 cloves garlic, minced ✓ 1/2 tbsp dried oregano	✓ 1/2 tsp salt ✓ Freshly cracked pepper ✓ To Serve: ✓ Rice or cauliflower rice ✓ Roasted vegetables, such as carrots, asparagus, or green beans	❖ In a large Ziplock bag or dish, add in the olive oil, lemon juice, garlic, oregano, salt, and pepper. Close the bag and shake the ingredients to combine, or stir the ingredients in the dish until well combined ❖ Filet each chicken breast into two thinner pieces and place the pieces in the bag or dish - make sure the chicken is completely covered in marinade and allow to marinate for up to minutes up to 8 hours, turn occasionally to maximize the marinade flavors. Once ready, heat a large skillet over medium heat ❖ Once heated, transfer the chicken from the marinade to the hot skillet and cook on each side cooked through, about 7 minutes each side, depending on the size - Discard of any excess marinade ❖ Transfer the cooked chicken from the skillet to a clean cutting board, allow to rest for five minutes before slicing ❖ Distribute the chicken, cooked rice and vegetables among the containers. Store in the fridge for up to 4 days. To Serve: Reheat in the microwave for 1-2 minutes or until heated through and enjoy!

Nutrition: Calories:446;Total Fat: 24g;Total Carbs: 4g;Fiber: 0g;Protein: 52g

77) TABOULI SALAD

		Cooking Time: 30 Minutes	Servings: 6

Ingredients	Ingredients	Instructions
✓ ½ cup extra fine bulgar wheat ✓ 4 firm Roma tomatoes, finely chopped, juice drained ✓ 1 English cucumber, finely chopped ✓ 2 bunches fresh parsley, stems removed, finely chopped	✓ 12-15 fresh mint leaves, finely chopped ✓ 4 green onions, finely chopped (white and green) ✓ salt ✓ 3-4 tbsp lime juice ✓ 3-4 tbsp extra virgin olive oil ✓ Romaine lettuce leaves ✓ pita bread	❖ Wash bulgur wheat thoroughly and allow it to soak under water for 5 minutes. ❖ Drain bulgur wheat well and set aside. ❖ Add all vegetables, green onions, and herbs to a dish. ❖ Add bulgur and season the mixture with salt. ❖ Add limejuice and olive oil. Mix well. ❖ Put to the jars and refrigerate. ❖ Transfer to a serving platter and serve with sides of pita and romaine lettuce.

78) ITALIAN-STYLE FLOUNDER

		Cooking Time: 45 Minutes	Servings: 4

Ingredients	Ingredients	Instructions
✓ Roma or plum tomatoes (5) ✓ Extra-virgin olive oil (2 tbsp.) ✓ Spanish onion (half of 1) ✓ Garlic (2 cloves) ✓ Italian seasoning (1 pinch) ✓ Kalamata olives (24)	✓ White wine (.25 cup) ✓ Capers (.25 cup) ✓ Lemon juice (1 tsp.) ✓ Chopped basil (6 leaves) ✓ Freshly grated parmesan cheese (3 tbsp.) ✓ Flounder fillets (1 lb.) ✓ Freshly torn basil (6 leaves)	❖ Set the oven to reach 425° Fahrenheit. Remove the pit and chop the olives (set aside. ❖ Pour water into a saucepan and bring to boiling. Plunge the tomatoes into the water and remove immediately. Add to a dish of ice water and drain. Remove the skins, chop, and set to the side for now. ❖ Heat a skillet with the oil using the medium temperature heat setting. Chop and toss in the onions. Sauté them for around four minutes. ❖ Dice and add the garlic, tomatoes, and seasoning. Simmer for five to seven minutes. ❖ Stir in the capers, wine, olives, half of the basil, and freshly squeezed lemon juice. ❖ Lower the heat setting and blend in the cheese. Simmer it until the sauce is thickened (15 min.. ❖ Arrange the flounder into a shallow baking tin. Add the sauce and garnish with the remainder of the basil leaves. ❖ Set the timer to bake it for 12 minutes until the fish is easily flaked.

Nutrition: Calories: 282;Protein: 24.4 grams;Fat: 15.4 grams

79) GREEK CHICKEN SOUP WITH LEMON

		Cooking Time: 20 Minutes	Servings: 8

Ingredients	Ingredients	Instructions
✓ 10 cups chicken broth ✓ 3 tbsp olive oil ✓ 8 cloves garlic, minced ✓ 1 sweet onion ✓ 1 large lemon, zested ✓ 2 boneless skinless chicken breasts	✓ 1 cup Israeli couscous (pearl) ✓ 1/2 tsp crushed red pepper ✓ 2 oz crumbled feta ✓ 1/3 cup chopped chive ✓ Salt, to taste ✓ Pepper, to taste	❖ In a large 6-8-quart sauce pot over medium-low heat, add the olive oil ❖ Once heated, sauté the onion and minced the garlic for 3-4 minutes to soften ❖ Then add in the chicken broth, raw chicken breasts, lemon zest, and crushed red pepper to the pot Raise the heat to high, cover, and bring to a boil ❖ Once boiling, reduce the heat to medium, then simmer for 5 minutes Stir in the couscous, 1 tsp salt, and black pepper to taste ❖ Simmer another 5 minute, then turn the heat off Using tongs, remove the two chicken breasts from the pot and transfer to a plate ❖ Use a fork and the tongs to shred the chicken, then return to the pot ❖ Stir in the crumbled feta cheese and chopped chive Season to taste with salt and pepper as needed ❖ Allow the soup to cool completely Distribute among the containers, store for 2-3 days ❖ To Serve: Reheat in the microwave for 1-2 minutes or until heated through, or reheat on the stove

80) ITALIAN-STYLE STEAMED SALMON WITH FRESH HERBS AND LEMON

	Cooking Time: 15 Minutes	Servings: 4

✓ 1 yellow onion, halved and sliced ✓ 4 green onions spring onions, trimmed and sliced lengthwise, divided ✓ 1 lb skin-on salmon fillet (such as wild Alaskan), cut into 4 portions ✓ 1/2 tsp Aleppo pepper ✓ 4 to 5 garlic cloves, chopped ✓ Extra virgin olive oil	✓ A large handful fresh parsley ✓ 1 lemon, thinly sliced ✓ 1 tsp ground coriander ✓ 1 tsp ground cumin ✓ 1/2 cup white wine (or you can use water or low-sodium broth, if you prefer) ✓ Kosher salt, to taste ✓ Black pepper, to taste	❖ Prepare a large piece of wax paper or parchment paper (about 2 feet long) and place it right in the center of a -inch deep pan or braiser ❖ Place the sliced yellow onions and a sprinkle a little bit of green onions the onions on the bottom of the braiser Arrange the salmon, skin-side down, on top, season with kosher salt and black pepper In a small bowl, mix together the coriander, cumin, and Aleppo pepper, coat top of salmon with the spice mixture, and drizzle with a little bit of extra virgin olive oil Then add garlic, parsley and the remaining green onions on top of the salmon (make sure that everything is arrange evenly over the salmon portions.) Arrange the lemon slices on top of the salmon Add another drizzle of extra virgin olive oil, then add the white wine Fold the parchment paper over to cover salmon, secure the edges and cover the braiser with the lid ❖ Place the braising pan over medium-high heat, cook for 5 minutes. Lower the heat to medium, cook for another 8 minutes, covered still. Remove from heat and allow to rest undisturbed for about 5 minutes. Remove the lid and allow the salmon to cool completely. Distribute among the containers, store for 2-3 days

81) BEEF SAUSAGE FRITTERS

	Cooking Time: 30 Minutes	Servings: 2

✓ 4 gluten-free Italian beef sausages, sliced ✓ 1 tbsp olive oil ✓ 1/3 large red bell peppers, seeded and sliced thinly ✓ 1/3 cup spinach	✓ ¾ tsp garlic powder ✓ 1/3 large green bell peppers, seeded and sliced thinly ✓ ¾ cup heavy whipped cream ✓ Salt and black pepper, to taste	❖ Mix together all the ingredients in a bowl except whipped cream and keep aside. Put butter and half of the mixture in a skillet and cook for about 6 minutes on both sides. Repeat with the remaining mixture and dish out. ❖ Beat whipped cream in another bowl until smooth. Serve the beef sausage pancakes with whipped cream. For meal prepping, it is compulsory to gently slice the sausages before mixing with other ingredients.

82) CARROT SOUP AND PARMESAN CROUTONS

	Cooking Time: 25 To 30 Minutes	Servings: 4

✓ 2 cups vegetable broth, no salt added, and low sodium is best ✓ 1 tsp dried thyme ✓ ¼ tsp sea salt ✓ 1 ounce grated parmesan cheese	✓ 2 pounds of carrots, unpeeled ✓ 2 tbsp extra virgin olive oil ✓ ½ chopped onion ✓ 2 ½ cups water ✓ ¼ tsp crushed red pepper ✓ 4 slices of whole-grain bread	❖ Cut your carrots into ½-inch slices. Take one rack from your oven and place it four inches from the broiler heating element. One either rack, place two large-rimmed baking sheets and turn your oven to 450 degrees Fahrenheit. Add 1 tbsp of oil and carrots into a large bowl. Stir the carrots around so they become coated with the oil. ❖ Using oven mitts, remove the baking pans and distribute the carrots onto them. Place the pans back into the oven and turn your timer on for 20 minutes or until the carrots become tender. Take the carrots out of the oven. Turn your oven to broiler mode. Set a large stockpot on your stove and turn the range to medium-high. Pour in the remaining olive oil and the onion. Let it cook for 5 minutes while stirring occasionally. ❖ Pour in the broth, thyme, water, crushed red pepper, and sea salt. Stir well. Let the mixture cook until the ingredients come to a boil. Once the carrots are done in the oven, add them to the pot. Remove the pot from the heat and carefully pour the soup into a blender. You will want to pour it in batches and remember to hold the lid of the blender with a rag and release the steam after 30 seconds, so it doesn't explode. ❖ Once all the soup is mixed, add it all back into the pot and turn the range heat to medium. Cook until the soup is warm again. Spread a piece of parchment paper on top of a baking sheet, set the four pieces of bread on the paper. Sprinkle cheese across the slices and set them on the top rack in your oven. Turn your oven to broil and let the slices of bread roast for a couple of minutes. Once the cheese is melted, remove the bread from the oven so they don't burn. Chop the bread into croutons. ❖ Divide the soup into serving bowls, add the croutons, and enjoy!

83) BAKED COD IN GREEK STYLE

	Cooking Time: 12 Minutes	Servings: 4

✓ 1 ½ lb Cod fillet pieces (4–6 pieces) ✓ 5 garlic cloves, peeled and minced ✓ 1/4 cup chopped fresh parsley leaves ✓ Lemon Juice Mixture: ✓ 5 tbsp fresh lemon juice ✓ 5 tbsp extra virgin olive oil	✓ 2 tbsp melted vegan butter ✓ For Coating: ✓ 1/3 cup all-purpose flour ✓ 1 tsp ground coriander ✓ 3/4 tsp sweet Spanish paprika ✓ 3/4 tsp ground cumin ✓ 3/4 tsp salt ✓ 1/2 tsp black pepper	❖ Preheat oven to 400 degrees F. In a bowl, mix together lemon juice, olive oil, and melted butter, set aside. In another shallow bowl, mix all-purpose flour, spices, salt and pepper, set next to the lemon bowl to create a station ❖ Pat the fish fillet dry, then dip the fish in the lemon juice mixture then dip it in the flour mixture, shake off excess flour ❖ In a cast iron skillet over medium-high heat, add 2 tbsp olive oil. Once heated, add in the fish and sear on each side for color, but do not fully cook (just couple minutes on each side), remove from heat ❖ With the remaining lemon juice mixture, add the minced garlic and mix ❖ Drizzle all over the fish fillets. Bake for 10 minutes, for until the it begins to flake easily with a fork ❖ allow the dish to cool completely. Distribute among the containers, store for 2-3 days. To Serve: Reheat in the microwave for 1-2 minutes or until heated through. Sprinkle chopped parsley. Enjoy!

84) SOLE FISH WITH PISTACHIO

	Cooking Time: 10 Minutes	Servings: 4

✓ 4 (5 ounces boneless sole fillets ✓ Salt and pepper as needed ✓ ½ cup pistachios, finely chopped	✓ Zest of 1 lemon ✓ Juice of 1 lemon ✓ 1 tsp extra virgin olive oil	❖ Pre-heat your oven to 350 degrees Fahrenheit ❖ Line a baking sheet with parchment paper and keep it on the side ❖ Pat fish dry with kitchen towels and lightly season with salt and pepper ❖ Take a small bowl and stir in pistachios and lemon zest ❖ Place sol on the prepped sheet and press 2 tbsp of pistachio mixture on top of each fillet. Drizzle fish with lemon juice and olive oil ❖ Bake for 10 minutes until the top is golden and fish flakes with a fork ❖ Serve and enjoy!

85) TOMATO SOUP WITH BEEF

	Cooking Time: 1 Hour	Servings: 6

✓ 1 pound lean ground beef ✓ 1 medium onion, chopped ✓ 1 large green pepper, chopped ✓ 2 minced garlic cloves ✓ 1 large tomato, chopped ✓ 2 tbsp tomato paste	✓ 2 tbsp all-purpose flour ✓ ¼ cup uncooked rice ✓ 2 tbsp fresh chopped parsley (additional for garnish) ✓ 4 cups beef broth ✓ 2 tbsp olive oil ✓ salt ✓ pepper	❖ Add oil to large pot and heat over medium heat. ❖ Add flour and keep whisking until thick paste forms. ❖ Keep whisking for 4 minutes while it bubbles and begins to thin. ❖ Add onions and sauté for 3-minutes. ❖ Stir in tomato paste and ground beef, breaking up ground beef with a wooden spoon. ❖ Cook for about 5 minutes. ❖ Add garlic, peppers, and tomatoes. ❖ Mix well until thoroughly combined. ❖ Add broth and bring the mixture to a light boil. ❖ Reduce heat to low, cover, and simmer for 30 minutes, making sure to stir from time to time. ❖ Add rice and parsley and cook for another 15 minutes. ❖ Once the soup has achieved its desired consistency, serve with a garnish of parsley. ❖ This soup is best enjoyed with some crispy bread or boiled potatoes.

86) BAKED TILAPIA

	Cooking Time: 15 Minutes	Servings: 4

Ingredients:

- ✓ 1 lb tilapia fillets (about 8 fillets)
- ✓ 1 tsp olive oil
- ✓ 1 tbsp vegan butter
- ✓ 2 shallots finely chopped
- ✓ 3 garlic cloves minced
- ✓ 1 1/2 tsp ground cumin
- ✓ 1 1/2 tsp paprika
- ✓ 1/4 cup capers
- ✓ 1/4 cup fresh dill finely chopped
- ✓ Juice from 1 lemon
- ✓ Salt & Pepper to taste

Directions:

- ❖ Preheat oven to 375 degrees F
- ❖ Line a rimmed baking sheet with parchment paper or foil
- ❖ Lightly mist with cooking spray, arrange the fish fillets evenly on baking sheet
- ❖ In a small bowl, combine the cumin, paprika, salt and pepper
- ❖ Season both sides of the fish fillets with the spice mixture
- ❖ In a small bowl, whisk together the melted butter, lemon juice, shallots, olive oil, and garlic, and brush evenly over fish fillets
- ❖ Top with the capers
- ❖ Bake in the oven for 10-15 minutes, until cook through, but not overcooked
- ❖ Remove from oven and allow the dish to cool completely
- ❖ Distribute among the containers, store for 2-3 days
- ❖ To Serve: Reheat in the microwave for 1-2 minutes or until heated through. Top with fresh dill. Serve!

87) HERBAL LAMB CUTLETS AND ROASTED VEGGIES

	Cooking Time: 45 Minutes	Servings: 6

Ingredients:

- ✓ 2 deseeded peppers, cut up into chunks
- ✓ 1 large sweet potato, peeled and chopped
- ✓ 2 sliced courgettes
- ✓ 1 red onion, cut into wedges
- ✓ 1 tbsp olive oil
- ✓ 8 lean lamb cutlets
- ✓ 1 tbsp thyme leaf, chopped
- ✓ 2 tbsp mint leaves, chopped

Directions:

- ❖ Preheat oven to 390degrees F.
- ❖ In a large baking dish, place peppers, courgettes, sweet potatoes, and onion.
- ❖ Drizzle all with oil and season with ground pepper.
- ❖ Roast for about 25 minutes
- ❖ Trim as much fat off the lamb as possible.
- ❖ Mix in herbs with a few twists of ground black pepper.
- ❖ Take the veggies out of the oven and push to one side of a baking dish.
- ❖ Place lamb cutlets on another side, return to oven, and roast for another 10 minutes.
- ❖ Turn the cutlets over, cook for another 10 minutes, and until the veggies are ready (lightly charred and tender).
- ❖ Mix everything on the tray and spread over containers.

Nutrition: Calories: 268, Total Fat: 9.2 g, Saturated Fat: 3 g, Cholesterol: 100 mg, Sodium: mg, Total Carbohydrate: 10.7 g, Dietary Fiber: 2.4 g, Total Sugars: 4.1 g, Protein: 32.4 g, Vitamin D: 0 mcg, Calcium: 20 mg, Iron: 4 mg, Potassium: 365 mg

88) WONDERFUL DENTEX ALLA MEDITERRANEA

	Cooking Time: 10 Minutes	**Servings: 2**

✓ 2 tbsp extra virgin olive oil ✓ 1 medium onion, chopped ✓ 2 garlic cloves, minced ✓ 1 tsp oregano ✓ 1 can (14 ounces tomatoes, diced with juice	✓ ½ cup black olives, sliced ✓ 4 red snapper fillets (each 4 ounce ✓ Salt and pepper as needed ✓ Garnish ✓ ¼ cup feta cheese, crumbled ✓ ¼ cup parsley, minced	❖ Pre-heat your oven to a temperature of 425-degree Fahrenheit ❖ Take a 13x9 inch baking dish and grease it up with non-stick cooking spray ❖ Take a large sized skillet and place it over medium heat ❖ Add oil and heat it up ❖ Add onion, oregano and garlic ❖ Saute for 2 minutes ❖ Add diced tomatoes with juice alongside black olives ❖ Bring the mix to a boil ❖ Remove the heat ❖ Place the fish on the prepped baking dish ❖ Season both sides with salt and pepper ❖ Spoon the tomato mix over the fish ❖ Bake for 10 minutes ❖ Remove the oven and sprinkle a bit of parsley and feta ❖ Enjoy! ❖ Meal Prep/Storage Options: Store in airtight containers in your fridge for 1-3 days

89) ITALIAN-STYLE PASTA SALAD

	Cooking Time: 25 Minutes	**Servings: 8**

✓ Salad: ✓ 8 oz pasta, I used farfalle, any smallish pasta works great! ✓ 1 cup rotisserie chicken, chopped ✓ 1/2 cup sun-dried tomatoes packed in oil, drained and coarsely chopped ✓ 1/2 cup jarred marinated artichoke hearts, drained and coarsely chopped ✓ 1/2 of 1 full English cucumber, chopped ✓ 1/3 cup kalamata olives, coarsely chopped ✓ 2 cups lightly packed fresh arugula ✓ 1/4 cup fresh flat leaf Italian parsley, coarsely chopped ✓ 1 small avocado, pit removed and coarsely chopped ✓ 1/3 cup feta cheese	✓ Dressing: ✓ 4 tbsp red wine vinegar ✓ 1 ½ tbsp ✓ dijon mustard, do not use regular mustard ✓ 1/2 tsp dried oregano ✓ 1 tsp dried basil ✓ 1 clove garlic, minced ✓ 1-2 tsp honey ✓ 1/2 cup olive oil ✓ 3 tbsp freshly squeezed lemon juice ✓ Fine sea salt, to taste ✓ Freshly cracked pepper, to taste	❖ Prepare the pasta according to package directions until al dente, drain the pasta and allow it to completely cool to room temperature, then add it to a large bowl ❖ Add in the chopped rotisserie chicken, chopped cucumber, coarsely chopped kalamata olives, coarsely chopped sun-dried tomatoes, coarsely chopped artichoke hearts, arugula, and parsley, toss ❖ Distribute the salad among the containers, store for 2-days ❖ Prepare the dressing - In a mason jar with a lid, combine the red wine vinegar, Dijon mustard, garlic, 1/2 tsp salt (or to taste), dried oregano, dried basil and 1/tsp pepper (or to taste, honey (add to sweetness preference), olive oil, and freshly squeezed lemon juice, place the lid on the mason jar and shake to combine, store in fridge ❖ To Serve: Add in the avocado and feta cheese to the salad, drizzle with the dressing, adjust any seasonings salt and pepper to taste, serve

Nutrition: Calories:32Carbs: 24g;Total Fat: 21g;Protein: 8g

90) AVOCADO LEMON HERB CHICKEN SALAD

	Cooking Time: 15 Minutes	**Servings: 4**

✓ Marinade/ Dressing: ✓ 2 tbsp olive oil ✓ 1/4 cup fresh lemon juice ✓ 2 tbsp water ✓ 2 tbsp fresh chopped parsley ✓ 2 tsp garlic, minced ✓ 1 tsp each dried thyme and dried rosemary ✓ 1 tsp salt ✓ 1/4 tsp cracked pepper, or to taste	✓ 1 pound skinless & boneless chicken thigh fillets or chicken breasts ✓ Salad: ✓ 4 cups Romaine lettuce leaves, washed and dried ✓ 1 large avocado, pitted, peeled and sliced ✓ 8 oz feta cheese ✓ 1 cup grape tomatoes, halved ✓ 1/4 of a red onion, sliced, optional ✓ 1/4 cup diced bacon, trimmed of rind and fat (optional) ✓ Lemon wedges, to serve	❖ In a large jug, whisk together the olive oil, lemon juice, water, chopped parsley, garlic, thyme, rosemary, salt, and pepper ❖ Pour half of the marinade into a large, shallow dish and refrigerate the remaining marinade to use as the dressing ❖ Add the chicken to the marinade in the bowl, allow the chicken to marinate for 15- minutes (or up to two hours in the refrigerator if you can) ❖ In the meantime, ❖ Once the chicken is ready, place a skillet or grill over medium-high heat add 1 tbsp of oil in, sear the chicken on both sides until browned and cooked through about 7 minutes per side, depending on thickness, and discard of the marinade ❖ Allow the chicken to rest for 5 minutes, slice and then allow the chicken to cool ❖ Distribute among the containers, and keep in the refrigerator ❖ To Serve: Reheat the chicken in the microwave for 30 seconds to 1 minutes. In a bowl, add the romaine lettuce, avocado, feta cheese, grape tomatoes, red onion and bacon, mix to combine. Arrange the chicken over salad. Drizzle the salad with the Untouched dressing. Serve with lemon wedges and enjoy!

Nutrition: Calories:378;Carbs: 6g;Total Fat: 22g;Protein: 31g

91) LEEKS, VEGETABLES AND POTATOES IN BRAISED PORK GREEK STYLE

	Cooking Time: 1 Hour 40 Minutes	**Servings: 4**

✓ 1 tbsp olive oil, plus 2 tsp ✓ 1¼ pounds boneless pork loin chops, fat cap removed and cut into 1-inch pieces ✓ 2 leeks, white and light green parts quartered vertically and thinly sliced ✓ 1 bulb fennel, quartered and thinly sliced ✓ 1 cup chopped onion ✓ 1 tsp chopped garlic ✓ 2 cups reduced-sodium chicken broth	✓ 1 tsp fennel seed ✓ 1 tsp dried oregano ✓ ½ tsp kosher salt ✓ 1 pound baby red potatoes, halved ✓ 1 bunch chard, including stems, chopped ✓ 2 tbsp freshly squeezed lemon juice	❖ Heat tbsp of oil in a soup pot or Dutch oven over medium-high heat. When the oil is shimmering, add the pork cubes and brown for about 6 minutes, turning the cubes over after 3 minutes. Remove the pork to a plate. ❖ Add the remaining tsp of oil to the same pot and add the leeks, fennel, onion, and garlic. Cook for 3 minutes. ❖ Pour the broth into the pan, scraping up any browned bits on the bottom. Add the fennel seed, oregano, and salt, and add the pork, plus any juices that may have accumulated on the plate. Make sure the pork is submerged in the liquid. Place the potatoes on top, then place the chard on top of the potatoes. ❖ Cover, turn down the heat to low, and simmer for 1½ hours, until the pork is tender. When the pork is done cooking, add the lemon juice. Taste and add more salt if needed. Cool. ❖ Scoop 2 cups of the mixture into each of 4 containers. ❖ STORAGE: Store covered containers in the refrigerator for up to 5 days.

Nutrition: Total calories: 3; Total fat: 13g; Saturated fat: 3g; Sodium: 1,607mg; Carbohydrates: 33g; Fiber: 8g; Protein: 34g

92) DELICIOUS BROCCOLI TORTELLINI SALAD

		Cooking Time: 20 To 25 Minutes	Servings: 12

Ingredients	Ingredients	Directions
✓ 1 cup sunflower seeds, or any of your favorite seeds ✓ 3 heads of broccoli, fresh is best! ✓ ½ cup sugar ✓ 20 ounces cheese-filled tortellini	✓ 1 onion ✓ 2 tsp cider vinegar ✓ ½ cup mayonnaise ✓ 1 cup raisins-optional	❖ Cut your broccoli into florets and chop the onion. ❖ Follow the directions to make the cheese-filled tortellini. Once they are cooked, drain and rinse them with cold water. ❖ In a bowl, combine your mayonnaise, sugar, and vinegar. Whisk well to give the ingredients a dressing consistency. ❖ In a separate large bowl, toss in your seeds, onion, tortellini, raisins, and broccoli. ❖ Pour the salad dressing into the large bowl and toss the ingredients together. You will want to ensure everything is thoroughly mixed as you'll want a taste of the salad dressing with every bite!

Nutrition: calories: 272, fats: 8.1 grams, carbohydrates: 38.grams, protein: 5 grams.

93) AVOCADO ARUGULA SALAD

		Cooking Time: 15 Minutes	Servings: 4

Ingredients	Ingredients	Directions
✓ 4 cups packed baby arugula ✓ 4 green onions, tops trimmed, chopped ✓ 1½ cups shelled fava beans ✓ 3 Persian cucumbers, chopped ✓ 2 cups grape tomatoes, halved ✓ 1 jalapeno pepper, sliced ✓ 1 avocado, cored, peeled, and roughly chopped	✓ lemon juice, 1½ lemons ✓ ½ cup extra virgin olive oil ✓ salt ✓ pepper ✓ 1 garlic clove, finely chopped ✓ 2 tbsp fresh cilantro, finely chopped ✓ 2 tbsp fresh mint, finely chopped	❖ Place the lemon-honey vinaigrette Ingredients: in a small bowl and whisk them well. ❖ In a large mixing bowl, add baby arugula, fava beans, green onions, tomatoes, cucumbers, and jalapeno. ❖ Divide the whole salad among four containers. ❖ Before serving, dress the salad with the vinaigrette and toss. ❖ Add the avocado to the salad. ❖ Enjoy!

94) ITALIAN SALAD OF SALMON AND AVOCADO

		Cooking Time: 10 Minutes	Servings: 4

Ingredients	Ingredients	Directions
✓ 1 lb skinless salmon fillets ✓ Marinade/Dressing: ✓ 3 tbsp olive oil ✓ 2 tbsp lemon juice fresh, squeezed ✓ 1 tbsp red wine vinegar, optional ✓ 1 tbsp fresh chopped parsley ✓ 2 tsp garlic minced ✓ 1 tsp dried oregano ✓ 1 tsp salt ✓ Cracked pepper, to taste	✓ Salad: ✓ 4 cups Romaine (or Cos) lettuce leaves, washed and dried ✓ 1 large cucumber, diced ✓ 2 Roma tomatoes, diced ✓ 1 red onion, sliced ✓ 1 avocado, sliced ✓ 1/2 cup feta cheese crumbled ✓ 1/3 cup pitted Kalamata olives or black olives, sliced ✓ Lemon wedges to serve	❖ In a jug, whisk together the olive oil, lemon juice, red wine vinegar, chopped parsley, garlic minced, oregano, salt and pepper ❖ Pour out half of the marinade into a large, shallow dish, refrigerate the remaining marinade to use as the dressing ❖ Coat the salmon in the rest of the marinade ❖ Place a skillet pan or grill over medium-high, add 1 tbsp oil and sear salmon on both sides until crispy and cooked through ❖ Allow the salmon to cool ❖ Distribute the salmon among the containers, store in the fridge for 2-3 days ❖ To Serve: Prepare the salad by placing the romaine lettuce, cucumber, roma tomatoes, red onion, avocado, feta cheese, and olives in a large salad bowl. Reheat the salmon in the microwave for 30seconds to 1 minute or until heated through. ❖ Slice the salmon and arrange over salad. Drizzle the salad with the remaining untouched dressing, serve with lemon wedges.

95) BLACK CABBAGE AND BEET SALAD

Cooking Time: 50 Minutes		**Servings: 6**

Ingredients	Ingredients	Directions
✓ 1 bunch of kale, washed and dried, ribs removed, chopped ✓ 6 pieces washed beets, peeled and dried and cut into ½ inches ✓ ½ tsp dried rosemary ✓ ½ tsp garlic powder ✓ salt ✓ pepper ✓ olive oil ✓ ¼ medium red onion, thinly sliced	✓ 1-2 tbsp slivered almonds, toasted ✓ ¼ cup olive oil ✓ Juice of 1½ lemon ✓ ¼ cup honey ✓ ¼ tsp garlic powder ✓ 1 tsp dried rosemary ✓ salt ✓ pepper	❖ Preheat oven to 400 degrees F. ❖ Take a bowl and toss the kale with some salt, pepper, and olive oil. ❖ Lightly oil a baking sheet and add the kale. ❖ Roast in the oven for 5 minutes, and then remove and place to the side. ❖ Place beets in a bowl and sprinkle with a bit of rosemary, garlic powder, pepper, and salt; ensure beets are coated well. ❖ Spread the beets on the oiled baking sheet, place on the middle rack of your oven, and roast for 45 minutes, turning twice. ❖ Make the lemon vinaigrette by whisking all of the listed Ingredients: in a bowl. ❖ Once the beets are ready, remove from the oven and allow it to cool. ❖ Take a medium-sized salad bowl and add kale, onions, and beets. ❖ Dress with lemon honey vinaigrette and toss well. ❖ Garnish with toasted almonds. ❖ Enjoy!

96) Special marinated tuna steak

Cooking Time: 15-20 Minutes		**Servings: 4**

Ingredients	Ingredients	Directions
✓ Olive oil (2 tbsp.) ✓ Orange juice (.25 cup) ✓ Soy sauce (.25 cup) ✓ Lemon juice (1 tbsp.) ✓ Fresh parsley (2 tbsp.)	✓ Garlic clove (1) ✓ Ground black pepper (.5 tsp.) ✓ Fresh oregano (.5 tsp.) ✓ Tuna steaks (4 - 4 oz. Steaks)	❖ Mince the garlic and chop the oregano and parsley. ❖ In a glass container, mix the pepper, oregano, garlic, parsley, lemon juice, soy sauce, olive oil, and orange juice. ❖ Warm the grill using the high heat setting. Grease the grate with oil. ❖ Add to tuna steaks and cook for five to six minutes. Turn and baste with the marinated sauce. ❖ Cook another five minutes or until it's the way you like it. Discard the remaining marinade.

97) PASTA WITH PRAWNS AND GARLIC

Cooking Time: 15 Minutes		**Servings: 4**

Ingredients	Ingredients	Directions
✓ 6 ounces whole wheat spaghetti ✓ 12 ounces raw shrimp, peeled and deveined, cut into 1-inch pieces ✓ 1 bunch asparagus, trimmed ✓ 1 large bell pepper, thinly sliced ✓ 1 cup fresh peas ✓ 3 garlic cloves, chopped	✓ 1 and ¼ tsp kosher salt ✓ ½ and ½ cups non-fat plain yogurt ✓ 3 tbsp lemon juice ✓ 1 tbsp extra-virgin olive oil ✓ ½ tsp fresh ground black pepper ✓ ¼ cup pine nuts, toasted	❖ Take a large sized pot and bring water to a boil ❖ Add your spaghetti and cook them for about minutes less than the directed package instruction ❖ Add shrimp, bell pepper, asparagus and cook for about 2- 4 minutes until the shrimp are tender ❖ Drain the pasta and the contents well ❖ Take a large bowl and mash garlic until a paste form ❖ Whisk in yogurt, parsley, oil, pepper and lemon juice into the garlic paste ❖ Add pasta mix and toss well ❖ Serve by sprinkling some pine nuts! ❖ Enjoy! ❖ Meal Prep/Storage Options: Store in airtight containers in your fridge for 1-3 days.

Nutrition: Calories: 406;Fat: 22g;Carbohydrates: 28g;Protein: 26g

98) SHRIMPS IN BUTTER AND PAPRIKA

	Cooking Time: 30 Minutes	Servings: 2

✓ ¼ tbsp smoked paprika ✓ 1/8 cup sour cream ✓ ½ pound tiger shrimps	✓ 1/8 cup butter ✓ Salt and black pepper, to taste	❖ Preheat the oven to 390 degrees F and grease a baking dish. ❖ Mix together all the ingredients in a large bowl and transfer into the baking dish. ❖ Place in the oven and bake for about 15 minutes. ❖ Place paprika shrimp in a dish and set aside to cool for meal prepping. Divide it in 2 containers and cover the lid. Refrigerate for 1-2 days and reheat in microwave before serving.

Nutrition: Calories: 330 ;Carbohydrates: 1.;Protein: 32.6g;Fat: 21.5g;Sugar: 0.2g;Sodium: 458mg

99) MOROCCAN FISH

	Cooking Time: 1 Hour 25 Minutes	Servings: 12

✓ Garbanzo beans (15 oz. Can) ✓ Red bell peppers (2) ✓ Large carrot (1) ✓ Vegetable oil (1 tbsp.) ✓ Onion (1) ✓ Garlic (1 clove) ✓ Tomatoes (3 chopped/14.5 oz can)	✓ Olives (4 chopped) ✓ Chopped fresh parsley (.25 cup) ✓ Ground cumin (.25 cup) ✓ Paprika (3 tbsp.) ✓ Chicken bouillon granules (2 tbsp.) ✓ Cayenne pepper (1 tsp.) ✓ Salt (to your liking) ✓ Tilapia fillets (5 lb.)	❖ Drain and rinse the beans. Thinly slice the carrot and onion. Mince the garlic and chop the olives. Discard the seeds from the peppers and slice them into strips. ❖ Warm the oil in a frying pan using the medium temperature setting. Toss in the onion and garlic. Simmer them for approximately five minutes. ❖ Fold in the bell peppers, beans, tomatoes, carrots, and olives. ❖ Continue sautéing them for about five additional minutes. ❖ Sprinkle the veggies with the cumin, parsley, salt, chicken bouillon, paprika, and cayenne. ❖ Stir thoroughly and place the fish on top of the veggies. ❖ Pour in water to cover the veggies. ❖ Lower the heat setting and cover the pan to slowly cook until the fish is flaky (about 40 min..

100) SARDINES WITH SALAD OF NIÇOISE INSPIRATION

	Cooking Time: 15 Minutes	Servings: 4

✓ 4 eggs ✓ 12 ounces baby red potatoes (about 12 potatoes) ✓ 6 ounces green beans, halved ✓ 4 cups baby spinach leaves or mixed greens ✓ 1 bunch radishes, quartered (about 1⅓ cups)	✓ 1 cup cherry tomatoes ✓ 20 kalamata or niçoise olives (about ⅓ cup) ✓ 3 (3.75-ounce) cans skinless, boneless sardines packed in olive oil, drained ✓ 8 tbsp Dijon Red Wine Vinaigrette	❖ Place the eggs in a saucepan and cover with water. Bring the water to a boil. As soon as the water starts to boil, place a lid on the pan and turn the heat off. Set a timer for minutes. ❖ When the timer goes off, drain the hot water and run cold water over the eggs to cool. Peel the eggs when cool and cut in half. ❖ Prick each potato a few times with a fork. Place them on a microwave-safe plate and microwave on high for 4 to 5 minutes, until the potatoes are tender. Let cool and cut in half. ❖ Place green beans on a microwave-safe plate and microwave on high for 1½ to 2 minutes, until the beans are crisp-tender. Cool. ❖ Place 1 egg, ½ cup of green beans, 6 potato halves, 1 cup of spinach, ⅓ cup of radishes, ¼ cup of tomatoes, olives, and 3 sardines in each of 4 containers. Pour 2 tbsp of vinaigrette into each of 4 sauce containers. ❖ STORAGE: Store covered containers in the refrigerator for up to 4 days.

101)   POMODORO LETTUCE SALAD

	Cooking Time: 15 Minutes	Servings: 6

✓ 1 heart of Romaine lettuce, chopped ✓ 3 Roma tomatoes, diced ✓ 1 English cucumber, diced ✓ 1 small red onion, finely chopped ✓ ½ cup curly parsley, finely chopped	✓ 2 tbsp virgin olive oil ✓ lemon juice, ½ large lemon ✓ 1 tsp garlic powder ✓ salt ✓ pepper	❖ Add all Ingredients: to a large bowl. ❖ Toss well and transfer them to containers. ❖ Enjoy!

102)   FLAX, BLUEBERRY, AND SUNFLOWER BUTTER BITES

	Cooking Time: 10 Minutes	Servings: 6

✓ ¼ cup ground flaxseed ✓ ½ cup unsweetened sunflower butter, preferably unsalted ✓ ⅓ cup dried blueberries ✓ 2 tbsp all-fruit blueberry preserves	✓ Zest of 1 lemon ✓ 2 tbsp unsalted sunflower seeds ✓ ⅓ cup rolled oats	❖ Mix all the ingredients in a medium mixing bowl until well combined. ❖ Form 1balls, slightly smaller than a golf ball, from the mixture and place on a plate in the freezer for about 20 minutes to firm up. ❖ Place 2 bites in each of 6 containers and refrigerate. ❖ STORAGE: Store covered containers in the refrigerator for up to 5 days. Bites may also be stored in the freezer for up to 3 months.

103)   SPECIAL DIJON RED WINE VINAIGRETTE

	Cooking Time: 5 Minutes	Servings: ½ Cup

✓ 2 tsp Dijon mustard ✓ 3 tbsp red wine vinegar ✓ 1 tbsp water	✓ ¼ tsp dried oregano ✓ ¼ tsp chopped garlic ✓ ⅛ tsp kosher salt ✓ ¼ cup olive oil	❖ Place the mustard, vinegar, water, oregano, garlic, and salt in a small bowl and whisk to combine. ❖ Whisk in the oil, pouring it into the mustard-vinegar mixture in a thin steam. ❖ Pour the vinaigrette into a container and refrigerate. ❖ STORAGE: Store the covered container in the refrigerator for up to 2 weeks. Allow the vinaigrette to come to room temperature and shake before serving.

104) DELICIOUS CREAMY KETO CUCUMBER SALAD

	Cooking Time: 5 Minutes	Servings: 2

✓ 2 tbsp mayonnaise ✓ Salt and black pepper, to taste	✓ 1 cucumber, sliced and quartered ✓ 2 tbsp lemon juice	❖ Mix together the mayonnaise, cucumber slices, and lemon juice in a large bowl. ❖ Season with salt and black pepper and combine well. ❖ Dish out in a glass bowl and serve while it is cold.

Nutrition: Calories: 8Carbs: 9.3g;Fats: 5.2g;Proteins: 1.2g;Sodium: 111mg;Sugar: 3.8g

105) CABBAGE SOUP WITH SAUSAGE AND MUSHROOMS

	Cooking Time: 1 Hour 10 Minutes	Servings: 6

Ingredients:	✓ 1 pound sausage, cooked and sliced ✓ Salt and black pepper, to taste	Directions:
✓ 2 cups fresh kale, cut into bite sized pieces ✓ 6.5 ounces mushrooms, sliced ✓ 6 cups chicken bone broth		❖ Heat chicken broth with two cans of water in a large pot and bring to a boil. ❖ Stir in the rest of the ingredients and allow the soup to simmer on low heat for about 1 hour. ❖ Dish out and serve hot.

Nutrition: Calories: 259;Carbs: ;Fats: 20g;Proteins: 14g;Sodium: 995mg;Sugar: 0.6g

106) CLASSIC MINESTRONE SOUP

	Cooking Time: 25 Minutes	Servings: 6

✓ 2 tbsp olive oil ✓ 3 cloves garlic, minced ✓ 1 onion, diced ✓ 2 carrots, peeled and diced ✓ 2 stalks celery, diced ✓ 1 1/2 tsp dried basil ✓ 1 tsp dried oregano ✓ 1/2 tsp fennel seed ✓ 6 cups low sodium chicken broth ✓ 1 (28-ounce can diced tomatoes	✓ 1 (16-ounce can kidney beans, drained and rinsed ✓ 1 zucchini, chopped ✓ 1 (3-inch Parmesan rind ✓ 1 bay leaf ✓ 1 bunch kale leaves, chopped ✓ 2 tsp red wine vinegar ✓ Kosher salt and black pepper, to taste ✓ 1/3 cup freshly grated Parmesan ✓ 2 tbsp chopped fresh parsley leaves	❖ Preheat olive oil in the insert of the Instant Pot on Sauté mode. ❖ Add carrots, celery, and onion, sauté for 3 minutes. ❖ Stir in fennel seeds, oregano, and basil. Stir cook for 1 minute. ❖ Add stock, beans, tomatoes, parmesan, bay leaf, and zucchini. ❖ Secure and seal the Instant Pot lid then select Manual mode to cook for minutes at high pressure. ❖ Once done, release the pressure completely then remove the lid. ❖ Add kale and let it sit for 2 minutes in the hot soup. ❖ Stir in red wine, vinegar, pepper, and salt. ❖ Garnish with parsley and parmesan. ❖ Enjoy.

107) SPECIAL SALAD OF KOMBU SEAWEED		
Cooking Time: 40 Minutes		**Servings: 6**
✓ 4 garlic cloves, crushed ✓ 1 pound fresh kombu seaweed, boiled and cut into strips	✓ 2 tbsp apple cider vinegar ✓ Salt, to taste ✓ 2 tbsp coconut aminos	❖ Mix together the kombu, garlic, apple cider vinegar, and coconut aminos in a large bowl. ❖ Season with salt and combine well. ❖ Dish out in a glass bowl and serve immediately.

108) TURKEY MEATBALL WITH DITALINI SOUP		
Cooking Time: 40 Minutes		**Servings: 4**
✓ meatballs: ✓ 1 pound 93% lean ground turkey ✓ 1/3 cup seasoned breadcrumbs ✓ 3 tbsp grated Pecorino Romano cheese ✓ 1 large egg, beaten ✓ 1 clove crushed garlic ✓ 1 tbsp fresh minced parsley ✓ 1/2 tsp kosher salt ✓ Soup: ✓ cooking spray ✓ 1 tsp olive oil ✓ 1/2 cup chopped onion ✓ 1/2 cup chopped celery	✓ 1/2 cup chopped carrot ✓ 3 cloves minced garlic ✓ 1 can (28 ounces diced San Marzano tomatoes ✓ 4 cups reduced sodium chicken broth ✓ 4 torn basil leaves ✓ 2 bay leaves ✓ 1 cup ditalini pasta ✓ 1 cup zucchini, diced small ✓ Parmesan rind, optional ✓ Grated parmesan cheese, optional for serving	❖ Thoroughly combine turkey with egg, garlic, parsley, salt, pecorino and breadcrumbs in a bowl. ❖ Make 30 equal sized meatballs out of this mixture. ❖ Preheat olive oil in the insert of the Instant Pot on Sauté mode. ❖ Sear the meatballs in the heated oil in batches, until brown. ❖ Set the meatballs aside in a plate. ❖ Add more oil to the insert of the Instant Pot. ❖ Stir in carrots, garlic, celery, and onion. Sauté for 4 minutes. ❖ Add basil, bay leaves, tomatoes, and Parmesan rind. ❖ Return the seared meatballs to the pot along with the broth. ❖ Secure and sear the Instant Pot lid and select Manual mode for 15 minutes at high pressure. Once done, release the pressure completely then remove the lid. Add zucchini and pasta, cook it for 4 minutes on Sauté mode. ❖ Garnish with cheese and basil. Serve.

109) NICE COLD AVOCADO AND MINT SOUP		
Cooking Time: 5 Minutes		**Servings: 2**
✓ 1 cup coconut milk, chilled ✓ 1 medium ripe avocado ✓ 1 tbsp lime juice	✓ Salt, to taste ✓ 20 fresh mint leaves	❖ Put all the ingredients into an immersion blender and blend until a thick mixture is formed. ❖ Allow to cool in the fridge for about 10 minutes and serve chilled.

110) CLASSIC SPLIT PEA SOUP		
Cooking Time: 30 Minutes		**Servings: 6**
✓ 3 tbsp butter ✓ 1 onion diced ✓ 2 ribs celery diced ✓ 2 carrots diced ✓ 6 oz. diced ham	✓ 1 lb. dry split peas sorted and rinsed ✓ 6 cups chicken stock ✓ 2 bay leaves ✓ kosher salt and black pepper	❖ Set your Instant Pot on Sauté mode and melt butter in it. ❖ Stir in celery, onion, carrots, salt, and pepper. ❖ Sauté them for 5 minutes then stir in split peas, ham bone, chicken stock, and bay leaves. Seal and lock the Instant Pot lid then select Manual mode for 15 minutes at high pressure. ❖ Once done, release the pressure completely then remove the lid. Remove the ham bone and separate meat from the bone. ❖ Shred or dice the meat and return it to the soup. Adjust seasoning as needed then serve warm. Enjoy.

111) BAKED FILLET OF SOLE ITALIAN STYLE

Cooking Time: 15 Minutes		Servings: 6

✓ 1 lime or lemon, juice of ✓ 1/2 cup extra virgin olive oil ✓ 3 tbsp unsalted melted vegan butter ✓ 2 shallots, thinly sliced ✓ 3 garlic cloves, thinly-sliced ✓ 2 tbsp capers ✓ 1.5 lb Sole fillet, about 10–12 thin fillets ✓ 1 tsp garlic powder	✓ 4–6 green onions, top trimmed, halved lengthwise ✓ 1 lime or lemon, sliced (optional) ✓ 3/4 cup roughly chopped fresh dill for garnish ✓ 1 tsp seasoned salt, or to your taste ✓ 3/4 tsp ground black pepper ✓ 1 tsp ground cumin	❖ Preheat over to 375-degree F. In a small bowl, whisk together olive oil, lime juice, and melted butter with a sprinkle of seasoned salt, stir in the garlic, shallots, and capers. In a separate small bowl, mix together the pepper, cumin, seasoned salt, and garlic powder, season the fish fillets each on both sides ❖ On a large baking pan or dish, arrange the fish fillets and cover with the buttery lime. Arrange the green onion halves and lime slices on top ❖ Bake in 375 degrees F for 10-15 minutes, do not overcook. Remove the fish fillets from the oven. Allow the dish to cool completely. Distribute among the containers, store for 2-3 days ❖ To Serve: Reheat in the microwave for 1-2 minutes or until heated through. Garnish with the chopped fresh dill. Serve with your favorite and a fresh salad

112) BAKED CHICKEN BREAST

Cooking Time: 50 Minutes		Servings: 2

✓ 2 skinless and boneless chicken breasts (about 8 ounces each) ✓ salt ✓ ground black pepper ✓ ¼ cup olive oil	✓ ¼ cup freshly squeezed lemon juice ✓ 1 garlic clove, minced ✓ ½ tsp dried oregano ✓ ¼ tsp dried thyme	❖ Preheat oven to a temperature of 400 degrees F. ❖ Season the chicken breasts carefully with salt and pepper on all sides. ❖ Place the chicken in a bowl. ❖ Take another bowl and add olive oil, lemon juice, oregano, garlic, and thyme. Mix well to make the marinade. ❖ Pour the marinade on top of chicken breasts and allow to marinate for 10 minutes. Set an oven rack about inches above the heat source. ❖ Place the chicken breasts into a baking pan and pour extra marinade on top. Bake for about 35-45 minutes until the center is no longer pink and the juices run clear. Move the baking dish to top rack and broil for about 5 minutes. Cool, spread over containers with some side dish and enjoy!

113) LEMON FISH GRILL

Cooking Time: 15 Minutes		Servings: 4

✓ ¼ tsp sea salt ✓ 3 to 4 lemons ✓ ¼ tsp ground black pepper	✓ 4 ounces any fish fillets, such as salmon or cod ✓ 1 tbsp olive oil	❖ Ensure that the fish fillets are dry. If you know or feel they are a bit damp, take a paper towel and pat them dry. ❖ Leave the fish fillets on the counter for 10 minutes so they can stand at room temperature. ❖ Turn on your grill to medium-high heat or set the temperature to 400 degrees Fahrenheit. Using nonstick cooking spray, coat the grill so the fish won't stick. Take one lemon and cut it in half. Set one of the halves aside and cut the remaining half into ¼-inch thick slices. ❖ Now, take the other half of the lemon and squeeze at least 1 tbsp of juice out into a small bowl. Add oil into the small bowl and whisk the ingredients together. Brush the fish with the lemon and oil mixture. Make sure you get both sides of the fish. ❖ Arrange the lemon slices on the grill in the shape of the fish, it might take about 3 to 4 slices for one fish. Place the fish on top of the lemon slices and grill the ingredients together. If you don't have a lid for your grill, cover it with a different lid that will fit or use aluminum foil. ❖ When the fish is about half-way done, turn it over so the other side is laying on top of the lemon slices. You will know the fish is done when it starts to look flaky and separates easily, which you can check by gently pressing a fork onto the fish.

114) BAKED BEANS ITALIAN STYLE

Cooking Time: 15 To 20 Minutes.	Servings: 6

Ingredients		Directions
✓ ½ cup chopped onion ✓ ¼ cup red wine vinegar ✓ ¼ tbsp ground cinnamon ✓ 15 ounces or 2 cans of great northern beans, do not drain	✓ 2 tsp extra virgin olive oil ✓ 12 ounces tomato paste, low sodium ✓ ½ cup water	❖ Turn a burner to medium heat and add oil to a saucepan. ❖ Add the onion and cook for 4 to 5 minutes. Stir well. ❖ Combine the vinegar, tomato paste, cinnamon, and water. Mix until all the ingredients are well combined. ❖ Switch the heat to a low setting. ❖ Using a colander, drain one can of beans and pour into the pan. ❖ Open the second can of beans and pour all of it, including the liquid, into the saucepan and stir. ❖ Continue to cook the beans for 10 minutes while stirring frequently. ❖ Serve and enjoy!

Nutrition: calories: 236, fats: 3 grams, carbohydrates: 42 grams, protein: 10 grams

115) POMODORO TILAPIA

Cooking Time: 15 Minutes	Servings: 4

Ingredients:		Directions:
✓ 3 tbsp sun-dried tomatoes packed in oil, drained (juice/oil reserved) and chopped ✓ 1 tbsp capers, drained ✓ 2 pieces tilapia	✓ 1 tbsp oil from sun-dried tomatoes ✓ 1 tbsp lemon juice ✓ 2 tbsp Kalamata olives, pitted and chopped	❖ Preheat oven to 375 degrees F. ❖ Add sun-dried tomatoes, capers, and olives to a bowl; stir well and set aside. ❖ Place the tilapia fillets side by side on a baking sheet. ❖ Drizzle with oil and lemon juice. ❖ Bake for about 10-1minutes. ❖ Check the fish after 10 minutes to see if they are flakey. ❖ Once done, top the fish with tomato mixture.

Nutrition: Calories: , Total Fat: 4.4 g, Saturated Fat: 0.8 g, Cholesterol: 28 mg, Sodium: 122 mg, Total Carbohydrate: 0.8 g, Dietary Fiber: 0.3 g, Total Sugars: 0.3 g, Protein: 10.7 g, Vitamin D: 0 mcg, Calcium: 16 mg, Iron: 1 mg, Potassium: 26 mg

116) LENTIL SOUP WITH CHICKEN

Cooking Time: 45 Minutes	Servings: 4

Ingredients:		Directions:
✓ 1 pound dried lentils ✓ 12 ounces boneless chicken thigh meat ✓ 7 cups water ✓ 1 small onion, diced ✓ 2 scallions, chopped ✓ ¼ cup chopped cilantro	✓ 3 cloves garlic ✓ 1 medium tomato, diced ✓ 1 tsp garlic powder ✓ 1 tsp cumin ✓ ¼ tsp oregano ✓ ½ tsp paprika ✓ ½ tsp kosher salt	❖ Add all of the listed Ingredients: to your Instant Pot. ❖ Set your pot to SOUP mode and cook for 30 minutes. ❖ Allow the pressure to release naturally. ❖ Take the chicken out and shred. ❖ Place the chicken back in the pot and stir. ❖ Pour to the jars. ❖ Enjoy!

117) ASPARAGUS WRAPPED WITH BACON

	Cooking Time: 30 Minutes	**Servings:** 2

Ingredients:

- ✓ 1/3 cup heavy whipping cream
- ✓ 2 bacon slices, precooked
- ✓ 4 small spears asparagus
- ✓ Salt, to taste
- ✓ 1 tbsp butter

Directions:

- ❖ Preheat the oven to 360 degrees F and grease a baking sheet with butter.
- ❖ Meanwhile, mix cream, asparagus and salt in a bowl.
- ❖ Wrap the asparagus in bacon slices and arrange them in the baking dish.
- ❖ Transfer the baking dish in the oven and bake for about 20 minutes.
- ❖ Remove from the oven and serve hot.
- ❖ Place the bacon wrapped asparagus in a dish and set aside to cool for meal prepping. Divide it in 2 containers and cover the lid. Refrigerate for about 2 days and reheat in the microwave before serving.

Nutrition: Calories: 204 ;Carbohydrates: 1.4g;Protein: 5.9g;Fat: 19.3g;Sugar: 0.5g;Sodium: 291mg

118) COOL ITALIAN-STYLE FISH

	Cooking Time: 30 Minutes	**Servings:** 8

- ✓ 6 ounces halibut fillets
- ✓ 1 tbsp Greek seasoning
- ✓ 1 large tomato, chopped
- ✓ 1 onion, chopped
- ✓ 5 ounces kalamata olives, pitted
- ✓ ¼ cup capers
- ✓ ¼ cup olive oil
- ✓ 1 tbsp lemon juice
- ✓ Salt and pepper as needed

- ❖ Pre-heat your oven to 350-degree Fahrenheit
- ❖ Transfer the halibut fillets on a large aluminum foil Season with Greek seasoning
- ❖ Take a bowl and add tomato, onion, olives, olive oil, capers, pepper, lemon juice and salt
- ❖ Mix well and spoon the tomato mix over the halibut Seal the edges and fold to make a packet Place the packet on a baking sheet and bake in your oven for 30-40 minutes Serve once the fish flakes off and enjoy!
- ❖ Meal Prep/Storage Options: Store in airtight containers in your fridge for 1-2 days.

119) FANCY LUNCHEON SALAD

	Cooking Time: 40 Minutes	**Servings:** 2

- ✓ 6-ounce cooked salmon, chopped
- ✓ 1 tbsp fresh dill, chopped
- ✓ Salt and black pepper, to taste
- ✓ 4 hard-boiled grass-fed eggs, peeled and cubed
- ✓ 2 celery stalks, chopped
- ✓ ½ yellow onion, chopped
- ✓ ¾ cup avocado mayonnaise

- ❖ Put all the ingredients in a bowl and mix until well combined.
- ❖ Cover with a plastic wrap and refrigerate for about 3 hours to serve.
- ❖ For meal prepping, put the salad in a container and refrigerate for up to days

Nutrition: Calories: 303 ;Carbohydrates: 1.7g;Protein: 10.3g;Fat: 30 ;Sugar: 1g;Sodium: 31g

120) BEEF SAUTEED WITH MOROCCAN SPICES AND BUTTERNUT SQUASH WITH CHICKPEAS

Cooking Time: 15 Minutes	**Servings: 4**

- ✓ 1 tbsp olive oil, plus 2 tsp
- ✓ 1 pound precut butternut squash cut into ½-inch cubes
- ✓ 3 ounces scallions, white and green parts chopped (1 cup)
- ✓ 1 tbsp water
- ✓ ¼ tsp baking soda
- ✓ ¾ pound flank steak, sliced across the grain into ⅛-inch thick slices
- ✓ ½ tsp garlic powder
- ✓ ¼ tsp ground ginger
- ✓ ¼ tsp turmeric

- ✓ ¼ tsp ground cumin
- ✓ ¼ tsp ground coriander
- ✓ ⅛ tsp cayenne pepper
- ✓ ⅛ tsp ground cinnamon
- ✓ ½ tsp kosher salt, divided
- ✓ 1 (14-ounce) can chickpeas, drained and rinsed
- ✓ ½ cup dried apricots, quartered
- ✓ ½ cup cilantro leaves, chopped
- ✓ 2 tsp freshly squeezed lemon juice
- ✓ 8 tsp sliced almonds

- ❖ Heat tbsp of oil in a 12-inch skillet. Once the oil is hot, add the squash and scallions, and cook until the squash is tender, about 10 to 12 minutes.
- ❖ Mix the water and baking soda together in a small prep bowl. Place the beef in a medium bowl, pour the baking-soda water over it, and mix to combine. Let it sit for 5 minutes.
- ❖ In a small bowl, combine the garlic powder, ginger, turmeric, cumin, coriander, cayenne, cinnamon, and ¼ tsp of salt, then add the mixture to the beef. Stir to combine.
- ❖ When the squash is tender, turn the heat off and add the remaining ¼ tsp of salt and the chickpeas, dried apricots, cilantro, and lemon juice to taste. Stir to combine. Place the contents of the pan in a bowl to cool.
- ❖ Clean out the skillet and heat the remaining 2 tsp of oil over high heat. When the oil is hot, add the beef and cook until it is no longer pink, about 2 to 3 minutes.
- ❖ Place 1¼ cups of the squash mixture and one quarter of the beef slices in each of 4 containers. Sprinkle 2 tsp of sliced almonds over each container.
- ❖ STORAGE: Store covered containers in the refrigerator for up to 5 days.

Nutrition: Total calories: 404; Total fat: 14g; Saturated fat: 1g; Sodium: 355mg; Carbohydrates: 46g; Fiber: 12g; Protein: 27g

121) NORTH AFRICAN–INSPIRED SAUTÉED SHRIMP AND LEEKS WITH PEPPERS

Cooking Time: 20 Minutes	**Servings: 4**

Ingredients:

- ✓ 2 tbsp olive oil, divided
- ✓ 1 large leek, white and light green parts, halved lengthwise, sliced ¼-inch thick
- ✓ 2 tsp chopped garlic
- ✓ 1 large red bell pepper, chopped into ¼-inch pieces
- ✓ 1 cup chopped fresh parsley leaves (1 small bunch)
- ✓ ½ cup chopped fresh cilantro leaves (½ small bunch)
- ✓ ¼ tsp ground cumin

- ✓ ¼ tsp ground coriander
- ✓ 1 tsp smoked paprika
- ✓ 1 pound uncooked peeled, deveined large shrimp (20 to 25 per pound), thawed if frozen, blotted with paper towels
- ✓ 1 tbsp freshly squeezed lemon juice
- ✓ ⅛ tsp kosher salt

Directions:

- ❖ Heat 2 tsp of oil in a -inch skillet over medium heat. Once the oil is hot, add the leeks and garlic and sauté for 2 minutes. Add the peppers and cook for 10 minutes, or until the peppers are soft, stirring occasionally.
- ❖ Add the chopped parsley and cilantro and cook for 1 more minute. Remove the mixture from the pan and place in a medium bowl.
- ❖ Mix the cumin, coriander, and paprika in a small prep bowl.
- ❖ Add 2 tsp of oil to the same skillet and increase the heat to medium-high. Add the shrimp in a single layer, sprinkle the spice mixture over the shrimp, and cook for about 2 minutes. Flip the shrimp over and cook for 1 more minute. Add the leek and herb mixture, stir, and cook for 1 more minute.
- ❖ Turn off the heat and add the remaining 2 tsp of oil and the lemon juice. Taste to see whether you need the salt. Add if necessary.
- ❖ Place ¾ cup of couscous or other grain (if using) and 1 cup of the shrimp mixture in each of 4 containers.
- ❖ STORAGE: Store covered containers in the refrigerator for up to 4 days.

122) Italian-style Chicken With Sweet Potato And Broccoli

	Cooking Time: 30 Minutes	Servings: 8

		Directions:
✓ 2 lbs boneless skinless chicken breasts, cut into small pieces	✓ Coarse sea salt, to taste	❖ Preheat the oven to 425 degrees F
✓ 5-6 cups broccoli florets	✓ Freshly cracked pepper, to taste	❖ Toss the chicken pieces with the Italian seasoning mix and a drizzle of olive oil, stir to combine then store in the fridge for about 30 minutes
✓ 3 tbsp Italian seasoning mix of your choice	✓ Toppings:	❖ Arrange the broccoli florets and sweet potatoes on a sheet pan, drizzle with the olive oil, sprinkle generously with salt
	✓ Avocado	❖ Arrange the chicken on a separate sheet pan
	✓ Lemon juice	❖ Bake both in the oven for 12-1minutes
✓ a few tbsp of olive oil	✓ Chives	❖ Transfer the chicken and broccoli to a plate, toss the sweet potatoes and continue to roast for another 15 minutes, or until ready
	✓ Olive oil, for serving	❖ Allow the chicken, broccoli, and sweet potatoes to cool
✓ 3 sweet potatoes, peeled and diced		❖ Distribute among the containers and store for 2-3 days
		❖ To Serve: Reheat in the microwave for 1 minute or until heated through, top with the topping of choice. Enjoy
		❖ Recipe Notes: Any kind of vegetables work will with this recipe! So, add favorites like carrots, brussels sprouts and asparagus.

Nutrition: Calories:222;Total Fat: 4.9g;Total Carbs: 15.3g;Protein: 28g

123) VEGETABLE SOUP

	Cooking Time: 20 Minutes	Servings: 6

Ingredients:		**Directions:**
✓ 1 15-ounce can low sodium cannellini beans, drained and rinsed	✓ 1 tbsp fresh thyme leaves, chopped	❖ Mash half of the beans in a small bowl using the back of a spoon and put it to the side.
	✓ 2 tsp fresh sage, chopped	❖ Add the oil to a large soup pot and place over medium-high heat.
✓ 1 tbsp olive oil	✓ ½ tsp salt	❖ Add carrots, onion, celery, garlic, zucchini, thyme, salt, pepper, and sage.
✓ 1 small onion, diced	✓ ¼ tsp freshly ground black pepper	❖ Cook well for about 5 minutes until the vegetables are tender.
✓ 2 carrots, diced		❖ Add broth and tomatoes and bring the mixture to a boil.
✓ 2 stalks celery, diced	✓ 32 ounces low sodium chicken broth	❖ Add beans (both mashed and whole) and spinach.
✓ 1 small zucchini, diced		❖ Cook for 3 minutes until the spinach has wilted.
✓ 1 garlic clove, minced	✓ 1 14-ounce can no-salt diced tomatoes, undrained	❖ Pour the soup into the jars.
	✓ 2 cups baby spinach leaves, chopped	❖ Before serving, top with parmesan.
	✓ 1/3 cup freshly grated parmesan	❖ Enjoy!

Nutrition: Calories: 359, Total Fat: 7.1 g, Saturated Fat: 2.7 g, Cholesterol: 10 mg, Sodium: 854 mg, Total Carbohydrate: 51.1 g, Dietary Fiber: 20 g, Total Sugars: 5.7 g, Protein: 25.8 g, Vitamin D: 0 mcg, Calcium: 277 mg, Iron: 7 mg, Potassium: 1497 mg

124) GREEK-STYLE CHICKEN WRAPS

	Cooking Time: 15 Minutes	Servings: 2

Ingredients:

- Greek Chicken Wrap Filling:
- 2 chicken breasts 14 oz, chopped into 1-inch pieces
- 2 small zucchinis, cut into 1-inch pieces
- 2 bell peppers, cut into 1-inch pieces
- 1 red onion, cut into 1-inch pieces
- 2 tbsp olive oil
- 2 tsp oregano
- 2 tsp basil
- 1/2 tsp garlic powder
- 1/2 tsp onion powder
- 1/2 tsp salt
- 2 lemons, sliced
- To Serve:
- 1/4 cup feta cheese crumbled
- 4 large flour tortillas or wraps

Directions:

- Pre-heat oven to 425 degrees F
- In a bowl, toss together the chicken, zucchinis, olive oil, oregano, basil, garlic, bell peppers, onion powder, onion powder and salt
- Arrange lemon slice on the baking sheet(s), spread the chicken and vegetable out on top (use 2 baking sheets if needed)
- Bake for 15 minutes, until veggies are soft and the chicken is cooked through Allow to cool completely
- Distribute the chicken, bell pepper, zucchini and onions among the containers and remove the lemon slices Allow the dish to cool completely
- Distribute among the containers, store for 3 days
- To Serve: Reheat in the microwave for 1-2 minutes or until heated through. Wrap in a tortila and sprinkle with feta cheese. Enjoy

125) GARBANZO BEAN SOUP

	Cooking Time: 20 Minutes	Servings: 4

- 14 ounces diced tomatoes
- 1 tsp olive oil
- 1 15-ounce can garbanzo beans
- salt
- pepper
- 2 sprigs fresh rosemary
- 1 cup acini di pepe pasta

- Take a large saucepan and add tomatoes and ounces of the beans.
- Bring the mixture to a boil over medium-high heat.
- Puree the remaining beans in a blender/food processor.
- Stir the pureed mixture into the pan.
- Add the sprigs of rosemary to the pan.
- Add acini de Pepe pasta and simmer until the pasta is soft, making sure to stir it from time to time.
- Remove the rosemary.
- Season with pepper and salt.
- Enjoy!

126) ITALIAN SALAD OF SPINACH AND BEANS

	Cooking Time: 30 Minutes	Servings: 4

- 15 ounces drained and rinsed cannellini beans
- 14 ounces drained, rinsed, and quartered artichoke hearts
- 6 ounces or 8 cups baby spinach
- 14 ½ ounces undrained diced tomatoes, no salt is best
- 1 tbsp olive oil and any additional if you prefer
- ¼ tsp salt
- 2 minced garlic cloves
- 1 chopped onion, small in size
- ¼ tsp pepper
- ⅛ tsp crushed red pepper flakes
- 2 tbsp Worcestershire sauce

- Place a saucepan on your stovetop and turn the temperature to medium-high.
- Let the pan warm up for a minute before you pour in the tbsp of oil. Continue to let the oil heat up for another minute or two.
- Toss in your chopped onion and stir so all the pieces are bathed in oil. Saute the onions for minutes.
- Add the garlic to the saucepan. Stir and saute the ingredients for another minute.
- Combine the salt, red pepper flakes, pepper, and Worcestershire sauce. Mix well and then add the tomatoes to the pan. Stir the mixture constantly for about minutes.
- Add the artichoke hearts, spinach, and beans. Saute and stir occasionally to get the taste throughout the dish. Once the spinach starts to wilt, take the salad off of the heat.
- Serve and enjoy immediately to get the best taste.

127) SPECIAL FRUIT SALAD WITH MINT AND ORANGE BLOSSOM WATER

	Cooking Time: 10 Minutes	Servings: 5

Ingredients:

- ✓ 3 cups cantaloupe, cut into 1-inch cubes
- ✓ 2 cups hulled and halved strawberries
- ✓ ½ tsp orange blossom water
- ✓ 2 tbsp chopped fresh mint

Directions:

- ❖ In a large bowl, toss all the ingredients together.
- ❖ Place 1 cup of fruit salad in each of 5 containers.
- ❖ STORAGE: Store covered containers in the refrigerator for up to 5 days.

Nutrition: Total calories: 52; Total fat: 1g; Saturated fat: <1g; Sodium: 10mg; Carbohydrates: 12g; Fiber: 2g; Protein: 1g

128) ROASTED BROCCOLI WITH RED ONIONS AND POMEGRANATE SEEDS

	Cooking Time: 20 Minutes	Servings: 5

Ingredients:

- ✓ 1 (12-ounce) package broccoli florets (about 6 cups)
- ✓ 1 small red onion, thinly sliced
- ✓ 2 tbsp olive oil
- ✓ ¼ tsp kosher salt
- ✓ 1 (5.3-ounce) container pomegranate seeds (1 cup)

Directions:

- ❖ Preheat the oven to 425°F and line 2 sheet pans with silicone baking mats or parchment paper.
- ❖ Place the broccoli and onion on the sheet pans and toss with the oil and salt. Place the pans in the oven and roast for minutes.
- ❖ After removing the pans from the oven, cool the veggies, then toss with the pomegranate seeds.
- ❖ Place 1 cup of veggies in each of 5 containers.
- ❖ STORAGE: Store covered containers in the refrigerator for up to days.

Nutrition: Total calories: 118; Total fat: ; Saturated fat: 1g; Sodium: 142mg; Carbohydrates: 12g; Fiber: 4g; Protein: 2g

129) DELICIOUS CHERMOULA SAUCE

	Cooking Time: 10 Minutes	Servings: 1 Cup

Ingredients:

- ✓ 1 cup packed parsley leaves
- ✓ 1 cup cilantro leaves
- ✓ ½ cup mint leaves
- ✓ 1 tsp chopped garlic
- ✓ ½ tsp ground cumin
- ✓ ½ tsp ground coriander
- ✓ ½ tsp smoked paprika
- ✓ ⅛ tsp cayenne pepper
- ✓ ⅛ tsp kosher salt
- ✓ 3 tbsp freshly squeezed lemon juice
- ✓ 3 tbsp water
- ✓ ½ cup extra-virgin olive oil

Directions:

- ❖ Place all the ingredients in a blender or food processor and blend until smooth.
- ❖ Pour the chermoula into a container and refrigerate.
- ❖ STORAGE: Store the covered container in the refrigerator for up to 5 days.

Nutrition: (¼ cup): Total calories: 257; Total fat: 27g; Saturated fat: ; Sodium: 96mg; Carbohydrates: 4g; Fiber: 2g; Protein: 1g

130) DEVILED EGG PESTO WITH SUN-DRIED TOMATOES

	Cooking Time: 15 Minutes	Servings: 5

Ingredients:	✓ 2 tbsp low-fat (2%) plain Greek yogurt	❖ Place the eggs in a saucepan and cover with water. Bring the water to a boil. As soon as the water starts to boil, place a lid on the pan and turn the heat off. Set a timer for minutes.
✓ 5 large eggs	✓ 5 tsp sliced sun-dried tomatoes	❖ When the timer goes off, drain the hot water and run cold water over the eggs to cool.
✓ 3 tbsp prepared pesto		❖ Peel the eggs, slice in half vertically, and scoop out the yolks. Place the yolks in a medium mixing bowl and add the pesto, vinegar, and yogurt. Mix well, until creamy.
✓ ¼ tsp white vinegar		❖ Scoop about 1 tbsp of the pesto-yolk mixture into each egg half. Top each with ½ tsp of sun-dried tomatoes.
		❖ Place 2 stuffed egg halves in each of separate containers.
		❖ STORAGE: Store covered containers in the refrigerator for up to 5 days.

131) WHITE BEAN WITH MUSHROOM DIP

	Cooking Time: 8 Minutes	Servings: 3 Cups

Ingredients:	✓ 1 tbsp fresh thyme leaves	❖ Heat 2 tsp of oil in a -inch skillet over medium-high heat. Once the oil is shimmering, add the mushrooms and sauté for 6 minutes. Add the garlic and thyme and continue cooking for 2 minutes.
✓ 2 tsp olive oil, plus 2 tbsp	✓ 2 (15.5-ounce) cans cannellini beans, drained and rinsed	❖ While the mushrooms are cooking, place the beans and lemon juice, the remaining tbsp of oil, and the salt in the bowl of a food processor. Add the mushrooms as soon as they are done cooking and blend everything until smooth. Scrape down the sides of the bowl if necessary and continue to process until smooth.
✓ 8 ounces button or cremini mushrooms, sliced	✓ 2 tbsp plus 1 tsp freshly squeezed lemon juice	❖ Taste and adjust the seasoning with lemon juice or salt if needed.
✓ 1 tsp chopped garlic	✓ ½ tsp kosher salt	❖ Scoop the dip into a container and refrigerate.
		❖ STORAGE: Store the covered container in the refrigerator for up to days. Dip can be frozen for up to 3 months.

132) SPICY SAUTÉED CABBAGE IN NORTH AFRICAN STYLE

	Cooking Time: 10 Minutes	Servings: 4

Ingredients:	✓ ½ tsp caraway seeds	Directions:
✓ 2 tsp olive oil	✓ ½ tsp ground cumin	❖ Heat the oil in a -inch skillet over medium-high heat. Once the oil is hot, add the cabbage and cook down for 3 minutes. Add the coriander, garlic powder, caraway seeds, cumin, salt, and chili flakes (if using) and stir to combine. Continue cooking the cabbage for about 7 more minutes.
✓ 1 small head green cabbage (about 1½ to 2 pounds), cored and thinly sliced	✓ ¼ tsp kosher salt	❖ Stir in the lemon juice and cool.
✓ 1 tsp ground coriander	✓ Pinch red chili flakes (optional—if you don't like heat, omit it)	❖ Place 1 heaping cup of cabbage in each of 4 containers.
✓ 1 tsp garlic powder	✓ 1 tsp freshly squeezed lemon juice	❖ STORAGE: Store covered containers in the refrigerator for up to 5 days.

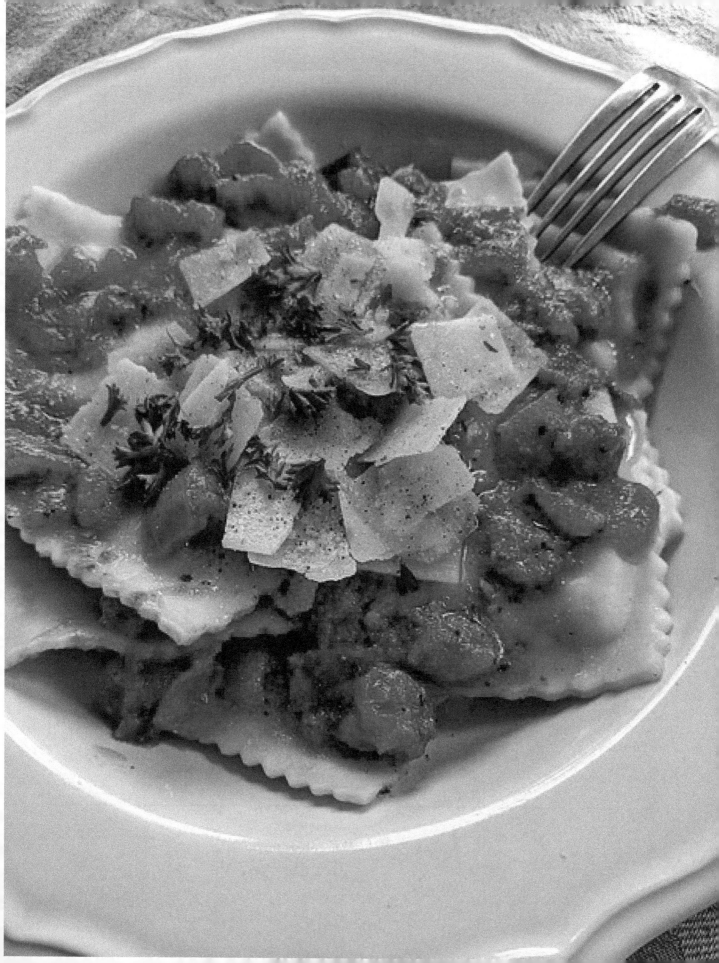

133) FLAX, BLUEBERRY, AND SUNFLOWER BUTTER BITES

	Cooking Time: 10 Minutes	Servings: 6

✓ ¼ cup ground flaxseed ✓ ½ cup unsweetened sunflower butter, preferably unsalted ✓ ⅓ cup dried blueberries ✓ 2 tbsp all-fruit blueberry preserves	✓ Zest of 1 lemon ✓ 2 tbsp unsalted sunflower seeds ✓ ⅓ cup rolled oats	❖ Mix all the ingredients in a medium mixing bowl until well combined. ❖ Form 1balls, slightly smaller than a golf ball, from the mixture and place on a plate in the freezer for about 20 minutes to firm up. ❖ Place 2 bites in each of 6 containers and refrigerate. ❖ STORAGE: Store covered containers in the refrigerator for up to 5 days. Bites may also be stored in the freezer for up to 3 months.

134) SPECIAL DIJON RED WINE VINAIGRETTE

	Cooking Time: 5 Minutes	Servings: ½ Cup

✓ 2 tsp Dijon mustard ✓ 3 tbsp red wine vinegar ✓ 1 tbsp water	✓ ¼ tsp dried oregano ✓ ¼ tsp chopped garlic ✓ ⅛ tsp kosher salt ✓ ¼ cup olive oil	❖ Place the mustard, vinegar, water, oregano, garlic, and salt in a small bowl and whisk to combine. ❖ Whisk in the oil, pouring it into the mustard-vinegar mixture in a thin steam. ❖ Pour the vinaigrette into a container and refrigerate. ❖ STORAGE: Store the covered container in the refrigerator for up to 2 weeks. Allow the vinaigrette to come to room temperature and shake before serving.

135) DELICIOUS CREAMY KETO CUCUMBER SALAD

	Cooking Time: 5 Minutes	Servings: 2

✓ 2 tbsp mayonnaise ✓ Salt and black pepper, to taste	✓ 1 cucumber, sliced and quartered ✓ 2 tbsp lemon juice	❖ Mix together the mayonnaise, cucumber slices, and lemon juice in a large bowl. ❖ Season with salt and black pepper and combine well. ❖ Dish out in a glass bowl and serve while it is cold.

Nutrition: Calories: 8Carbs: 9.3g;Fats: 5.2g;Proteins: 1.2g;Sodium: 111mg;Sugar: 3.8g

136) CABBAGE SOUP WITH SAUSAGE AND MUSHROOMS

	Cooking Time: 1 Hour 10 Minutes	Servings: 6

Ingredients: ✓ 2 cups fresh kale, cut into bite sized pieces ✓ 6.5 ounces mushrooms, sliced ✓ 6 cups chicken bone broth	✓ 1 pound sausage, cooked and sliced ✓ Salt and black pepper, to taste	**Directions:** ❖ Heat chicken broth with two cans of water in a large pot and bring to a boil. ❖ Stir in the rest of the ingredients and allow the soup to simmer on low heat for about 1 hour. ❖ Dish out and serve hot.

Nutrition: Calories: 259;Carbs: ;Fats: 20g;Proteins: 14g;Sodium: 995mg;Sugar: 0.6g

137)   CLASSIC MINESTRONE SOUP

	Cooking Time: 25 Minutes	Servings: 6

✓ 2 tbsp olive oil ✓ 3 cloves garlic, minced ✓ 1 onion, diced ✓ 2 carrots, peeled and diced ✓ 2 stalks celery, diced ✓ 1 1/2 tsp dried basil ✓ 1 tsp dried oregano ✓ 1/2 tsp fennel seed ✓ 6 cups low sodium chicken broth ✓ 1 (28-ounce can diced tomatoes	✓ 1 (16-ounce can kidney beans, drained and rinsed ✓ 1 zucchini, chopped ✓ 1 (3-inch Parmesan rind ✓ 1 bay leaf ✓ 1 bunch kale leaves, chopped ✓ 2 tsp red wine vinegar ✓ Kosher salt and black pepper, to taste ✓ 1/3 cup freshly grated Parmesan ✓ 2 tbsp chopped fresh parsley leaves	❖ Preheat olive oil in the insert of the Instant Pot on Sauté mode. ❖ Add carrots, celery, and onion, sauté for 3 minutes. ❖ Stir in fennel seeds, oregano, and basil. Stir cook for 1 minute. ❖ Add stock, beans, tomatoes, parmesan, bay leaf, and zucchini. ❖ Secure and seal the Instant Pot lid then select Manual mode to cook for minutes at high pressure. ❖ Once done, release the pressure completely then remove the lid. ❖ Add kale and let it sit for 2 minutes in the hot soup. ❖ Stir in red wine, vinegar, pepper, and salt. ❖ Garnish with parsley and parmesan. ❖ Enjoy.

138)   SPECIAL SALAD OF KOMBU SEAWEED

	Cooking Time: 40 Minutes	Servings: 6

✓ 4 garlic cloves, crushed ✓ 1 pound fresh kombu seaweed, boiled and cut into strips	✓ 2 tbsp apple cider vinegar ✓ Salt, to taste ✓ 2 tbsp coconut aminos	❖ Mix together the kombu, garlic, apple cider vinegar, and coconut aminos in a large bowl. ❖ Season with salt and combine well. ❖ Dish out in a glass bowl and serve immediately.

139)   TURKEY MEATBALL WITH DITALINI SOUP

	Cooking Time: 40 Minutes	Servings: 4

✓ meatballs: ✓ 1 pound 93% lean ground turkey ✓ 1/3 cup seasoned breadcrumbs ✓ 3 tbsp grated Pecorino Romano cheese ✓ 1 large egg, beaten ✓ 1 clove crushed garlic ✓ 1 tbsp fresh minced parsley ✓ 1/2 tsp kosher salt ✓ Soup: ✓ cooking spray ✓ 1 tsp olive oil ✓ 1/2 cup chopped onion ✓ 1/2 cup chopped celery	✓ 1/2 cup chopped carrot ✓ 3 cloves minced garlic ✓ 1 can (28 ounces diced San Marzano tomatoes ✓ 4 cups reduced sodium chicken broth ✓ 4 torn basil leaves ✓ 2 bay leaves ✓ 1 cup ditalini pasta ✓ 1 cup zucchini, diced small ✓ Parmesan rind, optional ✓ Grated parmesan cheese, optional for serving	❖ Thoroughly combine turkey with egg, garlic, parsley, salt, pecorino and breadcrumbs in a bowl. ❖ Make 30 equal sized meatballs out of this mixture. ❖ Preheat olive oil in the insert of the Instant Pot on Sauté mode. ❖ Sear the meatballs in the heated oil in batches, until brown. ❖ Set the meatballs aside in a plate. ❖ Add more oil to the insert of the Instant Pot. ❖ Stir in carrots, garlic, celery, and onion. Sauté for 4 minutes. ❖ Add basil, bay leaves, tomatoes, and Parmesan rind. ❖ Return the seared meatballs to the pot along with the broth. ❖ Secure and sear the Instant Pot lid and select Manual mode for 15 minutes at high pressure. ❖ Once done, release the pressure completely then remove the lid. ❖ Add zucchini and pasta, cook it for 4 minutes on Sauté mode. ❖ Garnish with cheese and basil. ❖ Serve.

140) NICE COLD AVOCADO AND MINT SOUP

	Cooking Time: 5 Minutes	Servings: 2

Ingredients:

- ✓ 1 cup coconut milk, chilled
- ✓ 1 medium ripe avocado
- ✓ 1 tbsp lime juice
- ✓ Salt, to taste
- ✓ 20 fresh mint leaves

Directions:

- ❖ Put all the ingredients into an immersion blender and blend until a thick mixture is formed.
- ❖ Allow to cool in the fridge for about 10 minutes and serve chilled.

141) CLASSIC SPLIT PEA SOUP

	Cooking Time: 30 Minutes	Servings: 6

Ingredients:

- ✓ 3 tbsp butter
- ✓ 1 onion diced
- ✓ 2 ribs celery diced
- ✓ 2 carrots diced
- ✓ 6 oz. diced ham
- ✓ 1 lb. dry split peas sorted and rinsed
- ✓ 6 cups chicken stock
- ✓ 2 bay leaves
- ✓ kosher salt and black pepper

Directions:

- ❖ Set your Instant Pot on Sauté mode and melt butter in it.
- ❖ Stir in celery, onion, carrots, salt, and pepper.
- ❖ Sauté them for 5 minutes then stir in split peas, ham bone, chicken stock, and bay leaves.
- ❖ Seal and lock the Instant Pot lid then select Manual mode for 15 minutes at high pressure.
- ❖ Once done, release the pressure completely then remove the lid.
- ❖ Remove the ham bone and separate meat from the bone.
- ❖ Shred or dice the meat and return it to the soup.
- ❖ Adjust seasoning as needed then serve warm.
- ❖ Enjoy.

142) BAKED FILLET OF SOLE ITALIAN STYLE

	Cooking Time: 15 Minutes	Servings: 6

Ingredients:

- ✓ 1 lime or lemon, juice of
- ✓ 1/2 cup extra virgin olive oil
- ✓ 3 tbsp unsalted melted vegan butter
- ✓ 2 shallots, thinly sliced
- ✓ 3 garlic cloves, thinly-sliced
- ✓ 2 tbsp capers
- ✓ 1.5 lb Sole fillet, about 10–12 thin fillets
- ✓ 4–6 green onions, top trimmed, halved lengthwise
- ✓ 1 lime or lemon, sliced (optional)
- ✓ 3/4 cup roughly chopped fresh dill for garnish
- ✓ 1 tsp seasoned salt, or to your taste
- ✓ 3/4 tsp ground black pepper
- ✓ 1 tsp ground cumin
- ✓ 1 tsp garlic powder

Directions:

- ❖ Preheat over to 375-degree F
- ❖ In a small bowl, whisk together olive oil, lime juice, and melted butter with a sprinkle of seasoned salt, stir in the garlic, shallots, and capers.
- ❖ In a separate small bowl, mix together the pepper, cumin, seasoned salt, and garlic powder, season the fish fillets each on both sides
- ❖ On a large baking pan or dish, arrange the fish fillets and cover with the buttery lime
- ❖ Arrange the green onion halves and lime slices on top
- ❖ Bake in 375 degrees F for 10-15 minutes, do not overcook
- ❖ Remove the fish fillets from the oven
- ❖ Allow the dish to cool completely
- ❖ Distribute among the containers, store for 2-3 days
- ❖ To Serve: Reheat in the microwave for 1-2 minutes or until heated through. Garnish with the chopped fresh dill. Serve with your favorite and a fresh salad
- ❖ Recipe Notes: If you can't get your hands on a sole fillet, cook this recipe with a different white fish. Just remember to change the baking time since it will be different.

Nutrition: Calories:350;Carbs:7 g;Total Fat: 26g;Protein: 23g

143) BAKED CHICKEN BREAST

	Cooking Time: 50 Minutes	Servings: 2

Ingredients	Ingredients	Directions
✓ 2 skinless and boneless chicken breasts (about 8 ounces each) ✓ salt ✓ ground black pepper ✓ ¼ cup olive oil	✓ ¼ cup freshly squeezed lemon juice ✓ 1 garlic clove, minced ✓ ½ tsp dried oregano ✓ ¼ tsp dried thyme	❖ Preheat oven to a temperature of 400 degrees F. ❖ Season the chicken breasts carefully with salt and pepper on all sides. ❖ Place the chicken in a bowl. ❖ Take another bowl and add olive oil, lemon juice, oregano, garlic, and thyme. Mix well to make the marinade. ❖ Pour the marinade on top of chicken breasts and allow to marinate for 10 minutes. Set an oven rack about inches above the heat source. ❖ Place the chicken breasts into a baking pan and pour extra marinade on top. Bake for about 35-45 minutes until the center is no longer pink and the juices run clear. Move the baking dish to top rack and broil for about 5 minutes. Cool, spread over containers with some side dish and enjoy!

144) LEMON FISH GRILL

	Cooking Time: 15 Minutes	Servings: 4

Ingredients	Ingredients	Directions
✓ ¼ tsp sea salt ✓ 3 to 4 lemons ✓ ¼ tsp ground black pepper	✓ 4 ounces any fish fillets, such as salmon or cod ✓ 1 tbsp olive oil	❖ Ensure that the fish fillets are dry. If you know or feel they are a bit damp, take a paper towel and pat them dry. ❖ Leave the fish fillets on the counter for 10 minutes so they can stand at room temperature. ❖ Turn on your grill to medium-high heat or set the temperature to 400 degrees Fahrenheit. Using nonstick cooking spray, coat the grill so the fish won't stick. Take one lemon and cut it in half. Set one of the halves aside and cut the remaining half into ¼-inch thick slices. ❖ Now, take the other half of the lemon and squeeze at least 1 tbsp of juice out into a small bowl. Add oil into the small bowl and whisk the ingredients together. Brush the fish with the lemon and oil mixture. Make sure you get both sides of the fish. ❖ Arrange the lemon slices on the grill in the shape of the fish, it might take about 3 to 4 slices for one fish. Place the fish on top of the lemon slices and grill the ingredients together. If you don't have a lid for your grill, cover it with a different lid that will fit or use aluminum foil. ❖ When the fish is about half-way done, turn it over so the other side is laying on top of the lemon slices. You will know the fish is done when it starts to look flaky and separates easily, which you can check by gently pressing a fork onto the fish.

145) BAKED BEANS ITALIAN STYLE

	Cooking Time: 15 To 20 Minutes.	Servings: 6

Ingredients	Ingredients	Directions
✓ ½ cup chopped onion ✓ ¼ cup red wine vinegar ✓ ¼ tbsp ground cinnamon ✓ 15 ounces or 2 cans of great northern beans, do not drain	✓ 2 tsp extra virgin olive oil ✓ 12 ounces tomato paste, low sodium ✓ ½ cup water	❖ Turn a burner to medium heat and add oil to a saucepan. ❖ Add the onion and cook for 4 to 5 minutes. Stir well. ❖ Combine the vinegar, tomato paste, cinnamon, and water. Mix until all the ingredients are well combined. ❖ Switch the heat to a low setting. ❖ Using a colander, drain one can of beans and pour into the pan. ❖ Open the second can of beans and pour all of it, including the liquid, into the saucepan and stir. ❖ Continue to cook the beans for 10 minutes while stirring frequently. ❖ Serve and enjoy!

Nutrition: calories: 236, fats: 3 grams, carbohydrates: 42 grams, protein: 10 grams

146) POMODORO TILAPIA

	Cooking Time: 15 Minutes	Servings: 4

Ingredients:

- ✓ 3 tbsp sun-dried tomatoes packed in oil, drained (juice/oil reserved) and chopped
- ✓ 1 tbsp capers, drained
- ✓ 2 pieces tilapia
- ✓ 1 tbsp oil from sun-dried tomatoes
- ✓ 1 tbsp lemon juice
- ✓ 2 tbsp Kalamata olives, pitted and chopped

Directions:

- ❖ Preheat oven to 375 degrees F.
- ❖ Add sun-dried tomatoes, capers, and olives to a bowl; stir well and set aside.
- ❖ Place the tilapia fillets side by side on a baking sheet.
- ❖ Drizzle with oil and lemon juice.
- ❖ Bake for about 10-1minutes.
- ❖ Check the fish after 10 minutes to see if they are flakey.
- ❖ Once done, top the fish with tomato mixture.

Nutrition: Calories: , Total Fat: 4.4 g, Saturated Fat: 0.8 g, Cholesterol: 28 mg, Sodium: 122 mg, Total Carbohydrate: 0.8 g, Dietary Fiber: 0.3 g, Total Sugars: 0.3 g, Protein: 10.7 g, Vitamin D: 0 mcg, Calcium: 16 mg, Iron: 1 mg, Potassium: 26 mg

147) LENTIL SOUP WITH CHICKEN

	Cooking Time: 45 Minutes	Servings: 4

Ingredients:

- ✓ 1 pound dried lentils
- ✓ 12 ounces boneless chicken thigh meat
- ✓ 7 cups water
- ✓ 1 small onion, diced
- ✓ 2 scallions, chopped
- ✓ ¼ cup chopped cilantro
- ✓ 3 cloves garlic
- ✓ 1 medium tomato, diced
- ✓ 1 tsp garlic powder
- ✓ 1 tsp cumin
- ✓ ¼ tsp oregano
- ✓ ½ tsp paprika
- ✓ ½ tsp kosher salt

Directions:

- ❖ Add all of the listed Ingredients: to your Instant Pot.
- ❖ Set your pot to SOUP mode and cook for 30 minutes.
- ❖ Allow the pressure to release naturally.
- ❖ Take the chicken out and shred.
- ❖ Place the chicken back in the pot and stir.
- ❖ Pour to the jars.
- ❖ Enjoy!

148) ASPARAGUS WRAPPED WITH BACON

	Cooking Time: 30 Minutes	Servings: 2

Ingredients:

- ✓ 1/3 cup heavy whipping cream
- ✓ 2 bacon slices, precooked
- ✓ 4 small spears asparagus
- ✓ Salt, to taste
- ✓ 1 tbsp butter

Directions:

- ❖ Preheat the oven to 360 degrees F and grease a baking sheet with butter.
- ❖ Meanwhile, mix cream, asparagus and salt in a bowl.
- ❖ Wrap the asparagus in bacon slices and arrange them in the baking dish.
- ❖ Transfer the baking dish in the oven and bake for about 20 minutes.
- ❖ Remove from the oven and serve hot.
- ❖ Place the bacon wrapped asparagus in a dish and set aside to cool for meal prepping. Divide it in 2 containers and cover the lid. Refrigerate for about 2 days and reheat in the microwave before serving.

Nutrition: Calories: 204 ;Carbohydrates: 1.4g;Protein: 5.9g;Fat: 19.3g;Sugar: 0.5g;Sodium: 291mg

149) COOL ITALIAN-STYLE FISH

Cooking Time: 30 Minutes		**Servings: 8**

Ingredients		Instructions
✓ 6 ounces halibut fillets ✓ 1 tbsp Greek seasoning ✓ 1 large tomato, chopped ✓ 1 onion, chopped ✓ 5 ounces kalamata olives, pitted	✓ ¼ cup capers ✓ ¼ cup olive oil ✓ 1 tbsp lemon juice ✓ Salt and pepper as needed	❖ Pre-heat your oven to 350-degree Fahrenheit ❖ Transfer the halibut fillets on a large aluminum foil Season with Greek seasoning ❖ Take a bowl and add tomato, onion, olives, olive oil, capers, pepper, lemon juice and salt ❖ Mix well and spoon the tomato mix over the halibut Seal the edges and fold to make a packet Place the packet on a baking sheet and bake in your oven for 30-40 minutes Serve once the fish flakes off and enjoy! ❖ Meal Prep/Storage Options: Store in airtight containers in your fridge for 1-2 days.

150) FANCY LUNCHEON SALAD

Cooking Time: 40 Minutes		**Servings: 2**

Ingredients		Instructions
✓ 6-ounce cooked salmon, chopped ✓ 1 tbsp fresh dill, chopped ✓ Salt and black pepper, to taste	✓ 4 hard-boiled grass-fed eggs, peeled and cubed ✓ 2 celery stalks, chopped ✓ ½ yellow onion, chopped ✓ ¾ cup avocado mayonnaise	❖ Put all the ingredients in a bowl and mix until well combined. ❖ Cover with a plastic wrap and refrigerate for about 3 hours to serve. ❖ For meal prepping, put the salad in a container and refrigerate for up to days

Nutrition: Calories: 303 ;Carbohydrates: 1.7g;Protein: 10.3g;Fat: 30g ;Sugar: 1g;Sodium: 31g

151) BEEF SAUTEED WITH MOROCCAN SPICES AND BUTTERNUT SQUASH WITH CHICKPEAS

Cooking Time: 15 Minutes		**Servings: 4**

Ingredients		Instructions
✓ 1 tbsp olive oil, plus 2 tsp ✓ 1 pound precut butternut squash cut into ½-inch cubes ✓ 3 ounces scallions, white and green parts chopped (1 cup) ✓ 1 tbsp water ✓ ¼ tsp baking soda ✓ ¾ pound flank steak, sliced across the grain into ⅛-inch thick slices ✓ ½ tsp garlic powder ✓ ¼ tsp ground ginger ✓ ¼ tsp turmeric	✓ ¼ tsp ground cumin ✓ ¼ tsp ground coriander ✓ ⅛ tsp cayenne pepper ✓ ⅛ tsp ground cinnamon ✓ ½ tsp kosher salt, divided ✓ 1 (14-ounce) can chickpeas, drained and rinsed ✓ ½ cup dried apricots, quartered ✓ ½ cup cilantro leaves, chopped ✓ 2 tsp freshly squeezed lemon juice ✓ 8 tsp sliced almonds	❖ Heat tbsp of oil in a 12-inch skillet. Once the oil is hot, add the squash and scallions, and cook until the squash is tender, about 10 to 12 minutes. ❖ Mix the water and baking soda together in a small prep bowl. Place the beef in a medium bowl, pour the baking-soda water over it, and mix to combine. Let it sit for 5 minutes. ❖ In a small bowl, combine the garlic powder, ginger, turmeric, cumin, coriander, cayenne, cinnamon, and ¼ tsp of salt, then add the mixture to the beef. Stir to combine. ❖ When the squash is tender, turn the heat off and add the remaining ¼ tsp of salt and the chickpeas, dried apricots, cilantro, and lemon juice to taste. Stir to combine. Place the contents of the pan in a bowl to cool. ❖ Clean out the skillet and heat the remaining 2 tsp of oil over high heat. When the oil is hot, add the beef and cook until it is no longer pink, about 2 to 3 minutes. ❖ Place 1¼ cups of the squash mixture and one quarter of the beef slices in each of 4 containers. Sprinkle 2 tsp of sliced almonds over each container. ❖ STORAGE: Store covered containers in the refrigerator for up to 5 days.

Nutrition: Total calories: 404; Total fat: 14g; Saturated fat: 1g; Sodium: 355mg; Carbohydrates: 46g; Fiber: 12g; Protein: 27g

152) NORTH AFRICAN–INSPIRED SAUTÉED SHRIMP AND LEEKS WITH PEPPERS

Cooking Time: 20 Minutes	Servings: 4

Ingredients:

- ✓ 2 tbsp olive oil, divided
- ✓ 1 large leek, white and light green parts, halved lengthwise, sliced ¼-inch thick
- ✓ 2 tsp chopped garlic
- ✓ 1 large red bell pepper, chopped into ¼-inch pieces
- ✓ 1 cup chopped fresh parsley leaves (1 small bunch)
- ✓ ½ cup chopped fresh cilantro leaves (½ small bunch)
- ✓ ¼ tsp ground cumin
- ✓ ¼ tsp ground coriander
- ✓ 1 tsp smoked paprika
- ✓ 1 pound uncooked peeled, deveined large shrimp (20 to 25 per pound), thawed if frozen, blotted with paper towels
- ✓ 1 tbsp freshly squeezed lemon juice
- ✓ ⅛ tsp kosher salt

Directions:

❖ Heat 2 tsp of oil in a -inch skillet over medium heat. Once the oil is hot, add the leeks and garlic and sauté for 2 minutes. Add the peppers and cook for 10 minutes, or until the peppers are soft, stirring occasionally.

❖ Add the chopped parsley and cilantro and cook for 1 more minute. Remove the mixture from the pan and place in a medium bowl.

❖ Mix the cumin, coriander, and paprika in a small prep bowl.

❖ Add 2 tsp of oil to the same skillet and increase the heat to medium-high. Add the shrimp in a single layer, sprinkle the spice mixture over the shrimp, and cook for about 2 minutes. Flip the shrimp over and cook for 1 more minute. Add the leek and herb mixture, stir, and cook for 1 more minute.

❖ Turn off the heat and add the remaining 2 tsp of oil and the lemon juice. Taste to see whether you need the salt. Add if necessary.

❖ Place ¾ cup of couscous or other grain (if using) and 1 cup of the shrimp mixture in each of 4 containers.

❖ STORAGE: Store covered containers in the refrigerator for up to 4 days.

153) Italian-style Chicken With Sweet Potato And Broccoli

Cooking Time: 30 Minutes	Servings: 8

- ✓ 2 lbs boneless skinless chicken breasts, cut into small pieces
- ✓ 5-6 cups broccoli florets
- ✓ 3 tbsp Italian seasoning mix of your choice
- ✓ a few tbsp of olive oil
- ✓ 3 sweet potatoes, peeled and diced
- ✓ Coarse sea salt, to taste
- ✓ Freshly cracked pepper, to taste
- ✓ Toppings:
- ✓ Avocado
- ✓ Lemon juice
- ✓ Chives
- ✓ Olive oil, for serving

Directions:

❖ Preheat the oven to 425 degrees F

❖ Toss the chicken pieces with the Italian seasoning mix and a drizzle of olive oil, stir to combine then store in the fridge for about 30 minutes

❖ Arrange the broccoli florets and sweet potatoes on a sheet pan, drizzle with the olive oil, sprinkle generously with salt

❖ Arrange the chicken on a separate sheet pan

❖ Bake both in the oven for 12-1minutes

❖ Transfer the chicken and broccoli to a plate, toss the sweet potatoes and continue to roast for another 15 minutes, or until ready

❖ Allow the chicken, broccoli, and sweet potatoes to cool

❖ Distribute among the containers and store for 2-3 days

❖ To Serve: Reheat in the microwave for 1 minute or until heated through, top with the topping of choice. Enjoy

❖ Recipe Notes: Any kind of vegetables work will with this recipe! So, add favorites like carrots, brussels sprouts and asparagus.

Nutrition: Calories:222;Total Fat: 4.9g;Total Carbs: 15.3g;Protein: 28g

154) VEGETABLE SOUP

	Cooking Time: 20 Minutes	Servings: 6

Ingredients:

- ✓ 1 15-ounce can low sodium cannellini beans, drained and rinsed
- ✓ 1 tbsp olive oil
- ✓ 1 small onion, diced
- ✓ 2 carrots, diced
- ✓ 2 stalks celery, diced
- ✓ 1 small zucchini, diced
- ✓ 1 garlic clove, minced
- ✓ 1 tbsp fresh thyme leaves, chopped
- ✓ 2 tsp fresh sage, chopped
- ✓ ½ tsp salt
- ✓ ¼ tsp freshly ground black pepper
- ✓ 32 ounces low sodium chicken broth
- ✓ 1 14-ounce can no-salt diced tomatoes, undrained
- ✓ 2 cups baby spinach leaves, chopped
- ✓ 1/3 cup freshly grated parmesan

Directions:

- ❖ Mash half of the beans in a small bowl using the back of a spoon and put it to the side.
- ❖ Add the oil to a large soup pot and place over medium-high heat.
- ❖ Add carrots, onion, celery, garlic, zucchini, thyme, salt, pepper, and sage.
- ❖ Cook well for about 5 minutes until the vegetables are tender.
- ❖ Add broth and tomatoes and bring the mixture to a boil.
- ❖ Add beans (both mashed and whole) and spinach.
- ❖ Cook for 3 minutes until the spinach has wilted.
- ❖ Pour the soup into the jars.
- ❖ Before serving, top with parmesan.
- ❖ Enjoy!

Nutrition: Calories: 359, Total Fat: 7.1 g, Saturated Fat: 2.7 g, Cholesterol: 10 mg, Sodium: 854 mg, Total Carbohydrate: 51.1 g, Dietary Fiber: 20 g, Total Sugars: 5.7 g, Protein: 25.8 g, Vitamin D: 0 mcg, Calcium: 277 mg, Iron: 7 mg, Potassium: 1497 mg

155) GREEK-STYLE CHICKEN WRAPS

	Cooking Time: 15 Minutes	Servings: 2

Ingredients:

- ✓ Greek Chicken Wrap Filling:
- ✓ 2 chicken breasts 14 oz, chopped into 1-inch pieces
- ✓ 2 small zucchinis, cut into 1-inch pieces
- ✓ 2 bell peppers, cut into 1-inch pieces
- ✓ 1 red onion, cut into 1-inch pieces
- ✓ 2 tbsp olive oil
- ✓ 2 tsp oregano
- ✓ 2 tsp basil
- ✓ 1/2 tsp garlic powder
- ✓ 1/2 tsp onion powder
- ✓ 1/2 tsp salt
- ✓ 2 lemons, sliced
- ✓ To Serve:
- ✓ 1/4 cup feta cheese crumbled
- ✓ 4 large flour tortillas or wraps

Directions:

- ❖ Pre-heat oven to 425 degrees F
- ❖ In a bowl, toss together the chicken, zucchinis, olive oil, oregano, basil, garlic, bell peppers, onion powder, onion powder and salt
- ❖ Arrange lemon slice on the baking sheet(s), spread the chicken and vegetable out on top (use 2 baking sheets if needed)
- ❖ Bake for 15 minutes, until veggies are soft and the chicken is cooked through Allow to cool completely
- ❖ Distribute the chicken, bell pepper, zucchini and onions among the containers and remove the lemon slices Allow the dish to cool completely
- ❖ Distribute among the containers, store for 3 days
- ❖ To Serve: Reheat in the microwave for 1-2 minutes or until heated through. Wrap in a tortila and sprinkle with feta cheese. Enjoy

Nutrition: (1 wrap): Calories:356;Total Fat: 14g;Total Carbs: 26g;Protein: 29g

156) GARBANZO BEAN SOUP		
	Cooking Time: 20 Minutes	Servings: 4

Ingredients	Ingredients	Instructions
✓ 14 ounces diced tomatoes ✓ 1 tsp olive oil ✓ 1 15-ounce can garbanzo beans	✓ salt ✓ pepper ✓ 2 sprigs fresh rosemary ✓ 1 cup acini di pepe pasta	❖ Take a large saucepan and add tomatoes and ounces of the beans. ❖ Bring the mixture to a boil over medium-high heat. ❖ Puree the remaining beans in a blender/food processor. ❖ Stir the pureed mixture into the pan. ❖ Add the sprigs of rosemary to the pan. ❖ Add acini de Pepe pasta and simmer until the pasta is soft, making sure to stir it from time to time. ❖ Remove the rosemary. ❖ Season with pepper and salt. ❖ Enjoy!

157) ITALIAN SALAD OF SPINACH AND BEANS		
	Cooking Time: 30 Minutes	Servings: 4

Ingredients	Ingredients	Instructions
✓ 15 ounces drained and rinsed cannellini beans ✓ 14 ounces drained, rinsed, and quartered artichoke hearts ✓ 6 ounces or 8 cups baby spinach ✓ 14 ½ ounces undrained diced tomatoes, no salt is best ✓ 1 tbsp olive oil and any additional if you prefer	✓ ¼ tsp salt ✓ 2 minced garlic cloves ✓ 1 chopped onion, small in size ✓ ¼ tsp pepper ✓ ⅛ tsp crushed red pepper flakes ✓ 2 tbsp Worcestershire sauce	❖ Place a saucepan on your stovetop and turn the temperature to medium-high. ❖ Let the pan warm up for a minute before you pour in the tbsp of oil. Continue to let the oil heat up for another minute or two. ❖ Toss in your chopped onion and stir so all the pieces are bathed in oil. Saute the onions for minutes. ❖ Add the garlic to the saucepan. Stir and saute the ingredients for another minute. ❖ Combine the salt, red pepper flakes, pepper, and Worcestershire sauce. Mix well and then add the tomatoes to the pan. Stir the mixture constantly for about minutes. ❖ Add the artichoke hearts, spinach, and beans. Saute and stir occasionally to get the taste throughout the dish. Once the spinach starts to wilt, take the salad off of the heat. ❖ Serve and enjoy immediately to get the best taste.

158)	SALMON SKILLET LUNCH	
	Cooking Time: 15 To 20 Minutes	**Servings: 4**

✓ 1 tsp minced garlic ✓ 1 ½ cup quartered cherry tomatoes ✓ 1 tbsp water ✓ ¼ tsp sea salt ✓ 1 tbsp lemon juice, freshly squeezed is best	✓ 1 tbsp extra virgin olive oil ✓ 12 ounces drained and chopped roasted red peppers ✓ 1 tsp paprika ✓ ¼ tsp black pepper ✓ 1 pound salmon fillets	❖ Remove the skin from your salmon fillets and cut them into 8 pieces. ❖ Turn your stove burner on medium heat and set a skillet on top. Pour the olive oil into the skillet and let it heat up for a couple of minutes. ❖ Add the minced garlic and paprika. Saute the ingredients for 1 minute. ❖ Combine the roasted peppers, black pepper, tomatoes, water, and salt. ❖ Set the heat to medium-high and bring the ingredients to a simmer. This should take 3 to 4 minutes. Remember to stir the ingredients occasionally so the tomatoes don't burn. Add the salmon and take some of the sauce from the skillet to spoon on top of the fish so it is all covered in the mixture. ❖ Cover the skillet and set a timer for 10 minutes. When the fish reaches 145 degrees Fahrenheit, it is cooked thoroughly. Turn off the heat and drizzle lemon juice over the fish. ❖ Break up the salmon into chunks and gently mix the pieces of fish with the sauce. Serve and enjoy!

159)	SALMON SKILLET LUNCH	
	Cooking Time: 15 To 20 Minutes	**Servings: 4**

✓ 1 tsp minced garlic ✓ 1 ½ cup quartered cherry tomatoes ✓ 1 tbsp water ✓ ¼ tsp sea salt ✓ 1 tbsp lemon juice, freshly squeezed is best	✓ 1 tbsp extra virgin olive oil ✓ 12 ounces drained and chopped roasted red peppers ✓ 1 tsp paprika ✓ ¼ tsp black pepper ✓ 1 pound salmon fillets	❖ Remove the skin from your salmon fillets and cut them into 8 pieces. ❖ Turn your stove burner on medium heat and set a skillet on top. Pour the olive oil into the skillet and let it heat up for a couple of minutes. ❖ Add the minced garlic and paprika. Saute the ingredients for 1 minute. ❖ Combine the roasted peppers, black pepper, tomatoes, water, and salt. ❖ Set the heat to medium-high and bring the ingredients to a simmer. This should take 3 to 4 minutes. Remember to stir the ingredients occasionally so the tomatoes don't burn. Add the salmon and take some of the sauce from the skillet to spoon on top of the fish so it is all covered in the mixture. ❖ Cover the skillet and set a timer for 10 minutes. When the fish reaches 145 degrees Fahrenheit, it is cooked thoroughly. Turn off the heat and drizzle lemon juice over the fish. ❖ Break up the salmon into chunks and gently mix the pieces of fish with the sauce. Serve and enjoy!

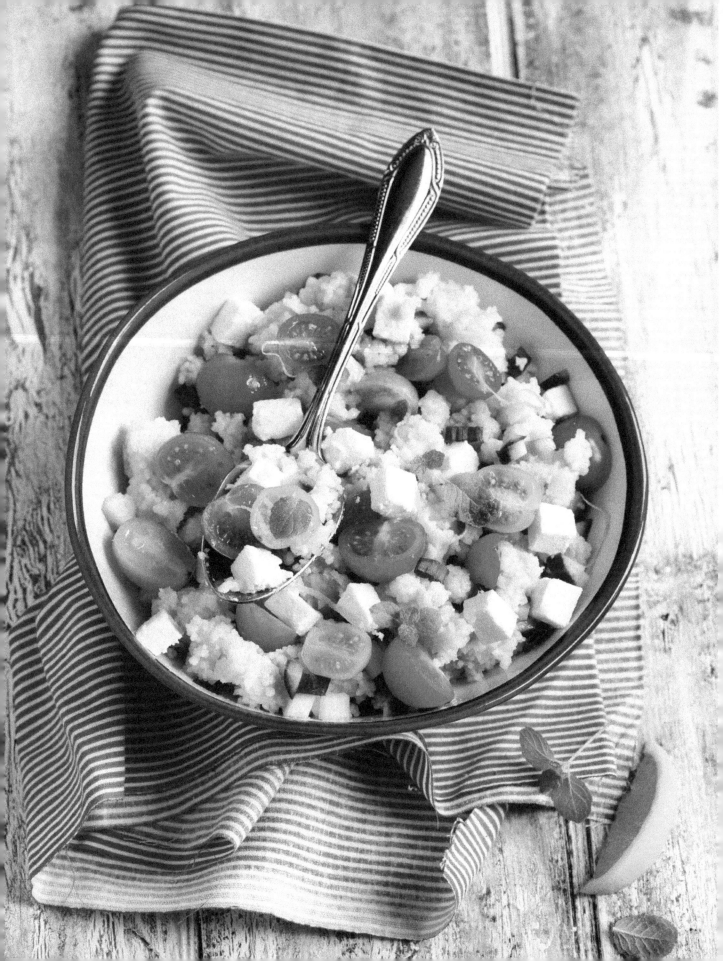

<u>Chapter 3.</u> DINNER

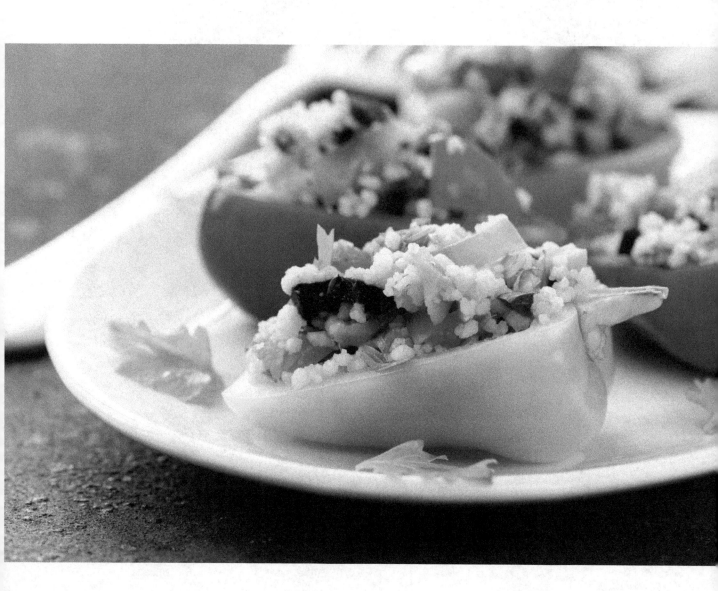

160) EASY ZUCCHINI SALAD WITH POMEGRANATE DRESSING

Preparation Time: 8 minutes	Cooking Time: 15 minutes	Servings: 6

Ingredients:

- ✓ One bunch of chives
- ✓ One pomegranate
- ✓ 1 tbsp pomegranate molasses
- ✓ 1/2 orange juice
- ✓ 1/4 cup mint leaf
- ✓ 120 g feta cheese
- ✓ 2 Lebanese cucumbers
- ✓ 2 tbsp currants
- ✓ 2 tbsp olive oil
- ✓ Three zucchinis
- ✓ salt and pepper

Directions:

- ❖ Clean the zucchini, then cucumber and slice the cucumber and cut it into ribbons using a peeler. And the same thing about your zucchini. Put the cucumber in the fridge.
- ❖ Chop chives into 2cm chunks and chop mint loosely.
- ❖ Make an orange Juice and combine with olive oil, a touch of pepper and salt, and 1 tbsp of pomegranate molasses to make the dressing. Whisk to blend.
- ❖ Toss the cucumber and zucchini into the dressing and apply the sliced herbs to prepare the salad.
- ❖ Add flowers and finish with the crumbled feta cheese.
- ❖ Slice the pomegranate into half and touch the skin's back with the dessert spoon to scatter the seeds over the salad.
- ❖ Now Serve.

Nutrition: Calories: 177.7 kcal Fat: 9.8 g Protein: 5.7 g Carbs: 20 g Fiber: 3.9 g

161) ITALIAN-STYLE GRAIN SALAD

Preparation Time: 5 minutes	Cooking Time: 35 minutes	Servings: 1

Ingredients:

- ✓ Coarse salt to taste
- ✓ Black pepper 2 tsp olive oil 1/2 minced small shallot 1/2 cup parsley, chopped 1
- ✓ 1 tbsp red wine vinegar 1 oz goat cheese, crumbled 1 cup grape tomatoes, halved

Directions:

- ❖ Combine the bulgur with 1/4 tsp salt and 1 cup of boiling water in a heat-proof dish. Cover, and let rest for about 30 minutes, before tender but somewhat chewy.
- ❖ Drain the bulgur and press to extract liquid in the fine-mesh sieve; return to the bowl. Add the onions, parsley, vinegar, shallot, and oil. Then season with pepper and salt, and toss.
- ❖ Top with cheese.

Nutrition: Calories:303 kcal Fat: 21g Protein: 10g Carbs: 21g Fiber: 4g

162) TROPICAL MACADAMIA NUTS DRESSING

Preparation Time: 10 minutes	Cooking Time: 10 minutes	Servings: 4

Ingredients:

- ✓ 1/4 tsp onion powder
- ✓ 1/2 tsp pepper
- ✓ 1 cup Cashew Milk
- ✓ 1 cup Macadamia Nuts
- ✓ 1 tbsp chives, chopped
- ✓ 1 tbsp lemon juice
- ✓ 1 tsp apple cider vinegar
- ✓ 1 tsp garlic powder
- ✓ 1 tsp salt
- ✓ 2 tbsp parsley

Directions:

- ❖ A high-powered mixer and places all the ingredients (other than green onions and chives, and parsley). Start at low and bring it up to high speed steadily until the ingredients are fully blended. If you want a thinner consistency, add more Homemade Cashew Milk from Nature's Eats.
- ❖ Add now the diced chives and parsley, then blend until smooth.
- ❖ Now serve promptly or store it in the refrigerator in an air-tight bag.

Nutrition: Calories: 302 kcal Fat: 26 g Protein: 8 g Carbs: 19 g Fiber: 6.3 g

163) EASY VINAIGRETTE DRESSING

Preparation Time: 5 minutes	Cooking Time: 5 minutes	Servings: 1

✓ black pepper, to taste ✓ 3 tbsp vinegar ✓ Two cloves garlic, minced	✓ 1 tbsp honey ✓ 1 tbsp Dijon mustard ✓ ½ cup olive oil ✓ ¼ tsp salt	❖ Combine all the ingredients in a liquid mixing cup. With a small spoon or a fork, stir well till ingredients are thoroughly mixed together. ❖ Now taste, and customize as needed. Thin it out with a little more olive oil if the mixture becomes too acidic, or balance the flavors with a bit more maple, honey, or syrup. Add a pinch of salt if the mixture is a bit blah. If the zing is not enough, apply a tsp of vinegar. ❖ Serve instantly, or for potential use, cover, and refrigerate. For 7 to 10 days, the homemade vinaigrette lasts well. If the vinaigrette solidifies in the fridge somewhat, don't think about it. It helps to do this with real olive oil. Simply let it for 5 to 10 minutes at room temperature or microwave very quickly (approximately 20 secs) to liquefy that olive oil again. Now serve.

164) Greek style turkey burger with Tzatziki sauce

Preparation Time: 36 minutes	Cooking Time: 10 minutes	Servings: 4

✓ Turkey Burgers ✓ 1 lb ground turkey ✓ 1/3 cup chopped sun-dried tomatoes ✓ ½ cup chopped spinach leaves ✓ 1/4 cup chopped red onion ✓ 2 pressed garlic cloves ✓ ¼ cup feta cheese ✓ One egg ✓ 1 tsp dried oregano ✓ 1 tbsp olive oil ✓ 1/2 tsp kosher salt ✓ One sliced red onion	✓ Four hamburger buns ✓ 1/2 tsp ground black pepper ✓ A handful of Bibb lettuce leaves ✓ Tzatziki Sauce ✓ ½ grated cucumber ✓ Two minced garlic cloves ✓ 3/4 cup Greek yogurt ✓ 1 tbsp red wine vinegar ✓ One pinch of kosher salt ✓ 1 tbsp chopped dill ✓ One pinch of black pepper	❖ Combine all the ingredients of Tzatziki sauce in a bowl and mix well. ❖ Mix turkey, onion, sun-dried tomatoes, and feta cheese in a bowl. ❖ In another bowl, mix olive oil, egg, garlic, salt, oregano, and pepper. ❖ Pour egg mixture with turkey mixture. Mix well. ❖ Make medium-sized patties out of turkey mixture. Set aside in the refrigerator for 24 hours. ❖ Cook turkey patties on heated grill sprayed with oil for seven minutes from both sides on medium flame. ❖ Spread Tzatziki sauce over buns and place lettuce, onions, and cooked patties and serve.

165) SAUCY GREEK-STYLE BAKED SHRIMP

Preparation Time: 15 minutes	Cooking Time: 20 minutes	Servings: 4

✓ 2 tbsp chopped dill ✓ 1 lb shrimp ✓ 1/4 tsp kosher salt ✓ 1/2 tsp red pepper flakes ✓ 3 tbsp olive oil ✓ Three minced garlic cloves	✓ One chopped onion ✓ 15 oz crushed tomatoes ✓ 1/2 tsp ground cinnamon ✓ 1/2 tsp ground allspice ✓ 1/2 cup crumbled feta cheese	❖ Add salt, shrimps, and pepper in a bowl. Toss well and keep it aside. ❖ Cook garlic and onions in heated olive oil over medium flame for five minutes. ❖ Add spices and stir for half a minute. ❖ Mix tomatoes and let it simmer for 20 minutes with occasional stirring. ❖ Transfer the tomato mixture to the baking sheet and add shrimps to it. Spread cheese and bake in a preheated oven at 375 degrees for 20 minutes. ❖ Drizzle dill and serve.

Nutrition: Calories: 190 kcal Fat: 5.2 g Protein: 25.9 g Carbs: 11.9 g Fiber: 5.2 g

166) TASTY SAUTÉED CHICKEN WITH OLIVES CAPERS AND LEMONS

Preparation Time: 5 minutes	Cooking Time: 30 minutes	Servings: 4

Ingredients:

- ✓ Six boneless chicken thighs
- ✓ Two sliced lemons
- ✓ One minced garlic clove minced
- ✓ 2/4 cup extra virgin olive oil
- ✓ 2 tbsp all-purpose flour
- ✓ 2 tbsp butter
- ✓ 1 cup chicken broth kosher salt to taste
- ✓ 3/4 cup Sicilian green olives
- ✓ 2 tbsp parsley
- ✓ 1/4 cup capers
- ✓ Black pepper to taste

Directions:

- ❖ Add salt, chicken, and pepper in a bowl and toss well. Set aside for 15 minutes.
- ❖ Cook lemon slices (half of them) in heated olive oil over medium flame for five minutes from both sides.
- ❖ Shift the cooked brown lemon slices on the plate.
- ❖ Coat chicken pieces with rice flour and cook in heated olive oil in the skillet for seven minutes from both sides. Transfer the cooked chicken to the plate.
- ❖ Sauté garlic in heated oil in the same pan for about half a minute. Stir in olives, chicken broth, lemons, and capers. Cook over high flame for few minutes.
- ❖ When half of the broth is left, add parsley and butter. Cook for one minute.
- ❖ Add salt and pepper to adjust the taste and serve.

Nutrition: Calories: 595 kcal Fat: 34 g Protein: 51 g Carbs: 5.5 g Fiber: 9 g

167) ENGLISH PORRIDGE (OATMEAL)

Preparation Time: 2 minutes	Cooking Time: 2 minutes	Servings: 1

Ingredients:

- ✓ Base Recipe
- ✓ ½ cup oats
- ✓ 1/2cup water
- ✓ 1/2cup milk
- ✓ 1 Pinch salt
- ✓ Maple Brown Sugar
- ✓ 1 tsp sugar
- ✓ 2 tbsp chopped pecans
- ✓ 1 tsp maple syrup
- ✓ 1/8 tsp cinnamon
- ✓ Banana Nut
- ✓ ½ banana sliced
- ✓ 1 tbsp flaxseed
- ✓ 2 tbsp walnuts
- ✓ 1/8 tsp cinnamon
- ✓ Strawberry & Cream
- ✓ 1/2cup strawberries
- ✓ 2 tsp honey
- ✓ 1 tbsp half and half
- ✓ 1/8 tsp vanilla extract
- ✓ Chocolate Peanut Butter
- ✓ 2 tsp cocoa powder
- ✓ 2 tsp chocolate chips
- ✓ 1 tbsp peanut butter
- ✓ 1 tsp roasted peanuts

Directions:

- ❖ Microwave Instructions
- ❖ Place all the ingredients heat in the microwave on high for 2 minutes. Then add 15-sec increments until the oatmeal is puffed and softened.
- ❖ Stovetop Instructions
- ❖ Bring the water and milk to a boil in a pan. Lower the heat & pour in the oats. Cook it while stirring, till the oats are soft and have absorbed most of the liquid.Turn off the stove and let it for 2 to 3 min.
- ❖ Assembly
- ❖ Stir in the toppings and let rest for a few minutes to cool. Serve warm.

Nutrition: Calories: 227 kcal Fat:6 g Protein: 9 g Carbs: 33 g Fiber: 4 g

168) MOROCCAN SALAD FATTOUSH

Preparation Time: 20 minutes	Cooking Time: 20 minutes	Servings: 6

Ingredients:

- ✓ Two loaves of pita bread
- ✓ • ½ tsp sumac
- ✓ • Olive Oil
- ✓ • Salt and pepper
- ✓ • One chopped English cucumber
- ✓ • One chopped lettuce
- ✓ • Five chopped Roma tomatoes
- ✓ Five radishes
- ✓ • Five chopped green onions
- ✓ • 2 cup parsley leaves
- ✓ Lime-vinaigrette
- ✓ • 1/4 tsp cinnamon
- ✓ • 1 tsp lime juice
- ✓ • Salt and pepper
- ✓ • 1/3 cup Virgin Olive Oil
- ✓ • 1 tsp sumac
- ✓ • 1/4 tsp allspice

Directions:

- ❖ Toast the bread in the oven. Heat olive oil and fry until browned. Add salt, pepper, and 1/2tsp of sumac. Turn off heat & place pita chips on paper towels to drain.
- ❖ In a mixing bowl, mix the chopped lettuce, cucumber, tomatoes, green onions with the sliced radish and parsley.
- ❖ For seasoning, whisk the lemon or lime juice, olive oil, and spices in a small bowl.
- ❖ Sprinkle the salad & toss lightly. Finally, add the pita chips and more sumac if you like. Shifts to small serving bowls or plates. Enjoy!

Nutrition: Calories: 345 kcal Fat:20.4 g Protein: 9.1 g Carbs:39.8 g Fiber: 1 g

169) CALABRIA CICORIA E FAGIOLI

Preparation Time:	Cooking Time:	Servings: 6

Ingredients:

- ✓ 200 g dried cannellini beans
- ✓ • 6 tbsp olive oil
- ✓ • 400 g curly endive
- ✓ Four garlic cloves
- ✓ • 600 ml of water
- ✓ • Two red chilies
- ✓ • Salt and pepper to taste

Directions:

- ❖ Put the dried beans to soak for 12 h (they increase in size). Drain them and boil for two h in fresh unsalted water. Salt at the end of the cooking time. If using canned beans, drain them from their liquid and rinse them before use. Rinse the endive and cut it up into short lengths.
- ❖ Heat the olive oil, fry the garlic without browning, and then add the endive and chilies. Keeping the heat high, stir-fry for a minute or two, coating the endive with the oil, then add the drained cannellini beans, some salt, and the water. Bring to the boil, cover the pan, and lower the heat. Cook until the endive is soft and most of the liquid has been absorbed.

Nutrition: Calories:225 kcal Fat: 21 g Protein: 3 g Carbs: 6 g Fiber:1 g

170)	CAMPANIA POACHED EGGS CAPRESE	
Preparation Time: 10 minutes	Cooking Time: 10 minutes	Servings: 2

Ingredients:

- ✓ 4 tsp pesto
- ✓ • 1 tbsp white vinegar
- ✓ • Four eggs
- ✓ • 2 tsp salt
- ✓ 2 English muffins
- ✓ • salt to taste
- ✓ • One tomato sliced
- ✓ • Four slices of mozzarella cheese

Directions:

- ❖ Fill 2 to 3 inches of a pan with water and boil over a high flame. Lower the heat, add the vinegar, 2 tsp of salt in it, and let it simmer.
- ❖ Put a cheese slice and a slice of tomato on every English muffin half and put in a toaster oven for 5 min or till the cheese melts and the English muffin is well toasted.
- ❖ Break an egg in a bowl and add in the water one by one. Let the eggs cook for 2.5 to 3 minutes or until the yolks have solidified and the egg whites are firm. Take the eggs out of the water and put them on a kitchen towel to absorb excess water.
- ❖ For assembling, first put an egg on top of every muffin, add a tsp of pesto sauce on the egg, and scatter the salt.

171)	GREEK BREAKFAST DISH WITH EGGS AND VEGETABLES	
Preparation Time: 10 minutes	Cooking Time: 10 minutes	Servings: 2

Ingredients:

- ✓ 1 tbsp olive oil
- ✓ • salt to taste
- ✓ • 2 cup chopped rainbow chard
- ✓ • ½ cup arugula
- ✓ 1 cup spinach
- ✓ • Two cloves garlic
- ✓ • ½ cup grated Cheddar cheese
- ✓ • Four eggs
- ✓ • black pepper to taste

Directions:

- ❖ Heat oil over moderate pressure. Sauté the chard, spinach, and arugula until soft, around three minutes. Add garlic, continue cooking until aromatic, approx. Two min.
- ❖ In a cup, combine the eggs and the cheese; dump into the mixture of the chard. Heat and cook for 5 - 6 minutes. Season to taste with salt and pepper.

172)	ITALIAN BREAKFAST PITA PIZZA	
Preparation Time: 25 minutes	Cooking Time: 30 minutes	Servings: 2

Ingredients:

- ✓ Four slices of bacon
- ✓ 2 tbsp olive oil
- ✓ 1/4 onion
- ✓ Four eggs
- ✓ Two pita bread rounds
- ✓ 2 tbsp pesto
- ✓ ½ tomato
- ✓ One avocado
- ✓ ½ cup slashed spinach
- ✓ 1/4 cup mushrooms
- ✓ ½ cup grated Cheddar cheese

Directions:

- ❖ Heat the oven to 350 ° F (175° C).
- ❖ In a medium saucepan, put the bacon and cook over medium-high heat, rotating periodically, when browned uniformly, around ten minutes. Cook the onion in the same skillet till smooth. Put it aside. In the skillet, melt the olive oil. Add the eggs and cook, stirring regularly, for 3 to 5 minutes.
- ❖ Add the pita bread to the cake pan. Cover with bacon, fried eggs, onions, mushrooms, and spinach; sprinkle the pesto over through the pita. Dress over the toppings of Cheddar cheese.
- ❖ Bake it in the preheated oven for 10 min. Serve with avocado pieces.

173) NAPOLI CAPRESE ON TOAST

Preparation Time: 15 minutes	Cooking Time: 5 minutes	Servings: 14

		Directions:
✓ 14 slices bread	✓ 3 tbsp olive oil	
✓ 1 lb mozzarella cheese	✓ Three tomatoes	❖ Baked the bread slices and spread the garlic on one side of each piece. Put a slice of mozzarella cheese, 1 to 2 basil leaves, and a slice of tomato on each piece of toast. Sprinkle with olive oil, spray salt, and black pepper.
✓ Two cloves garlic	✓ salt to taste	
✓ 1/3 cup basil leaves	✓ black pepper to taste	

Nutrition: Calories: 203.5 kcal Fat: 10 g Protein: 10.5 g Carbs: 16.5 g Fiber: 1.1 g

174) TUSCAN EGGS FLORENTINE

Preparation Time: 10 minutes	Cooking Time: 10 minutes	Servings: 3

Ingredients:	✓ ½ fresh spinach	Directions:
	✓ Salt to taste	
✓ 2 tbsp butter	✓ Six eggs	❖ Put the butter in a non-stick skillet; heat and mix the mushrooms and garlic till the garlic is flavorsome for about 1 min. Add spinach to the mushroom paste and cook until spinach is softened for 2 - 3 mins,
✓ Two cloves garlic	✓ Black pepper to taste	
✓ 3 tbsp cream cheese		❖ Mix the mushroom-spinach mixer; add salt and pepper. Cook, with mixing, until the eggs are stiff; turn. Pour with cream cheese over the egg mixture and cook before cream cheese started melting just over five minutes.
✓ ½ cup mushroom		

Nutrition: Calories: 278.9 kcal Fat: 22.9 g Protein:15.7 g Carbs: 4.1 g Fiber:22.9

175) SPECIAL QUINOA, CEREALS FOR BREAKFAST

Preparation Time: 5 minutes	Cooking Time: 16 minutes	Servings: 4

Ingredients:	✓ ½ cup almonds	Directions:
	✓ 1 tsp cinnamon	
✓ 2 cups of water	✓ 1/3 cup seeds	❖ Combine water and quinoa in a medium saucepan and continue cooking. Lower the heat and boil when much of the water has been drained for 8–12 minutes. Whisk in apricots, almonds, linseeds, cinnamon, and nutmeg; simmer till the quinoa is soft.
✓ ½ cup apricots	✓ ½ tsp nutmeg	
✓ 1 cup quinoa		

Nutrition: Calories: 349.9 kcal Fat:15.1 g Protein: 11.8 g Carbs: 44.5 g Fiber: 9.3 g

176) SIMPLE ZUCCHINI WITH EGG

Preparation Time: 5 minutes	Cooking Time: 15 minutes	Servings: 2

Ingredients:	✓ Two zucchinis	Directions:
	✓ Black pepper to taste	
✓ Two eggs	✓ 1 tsp water	❖ Heat the oil in a saucepan over medium heat; sauté the zucchini until soft, around 10 minutes. Season with salt and black pepper.
✓ 1.5 tbsp olive oil		❖ Add the eggs with a fork in a bowl; add more water and mix until uniformly mixed. Spill the eggs over the zucchini; continue cooking until the eggs are boiled and rubbery for almost 5 minutes. Dress it with salt and black pepper.
✓ salt to taste		

Nutrition: Calories: 21.7 kcal Fat: 15.7 g Protein: 10.2 g Carbs: 11.2 g Fiber: 3.6 g

177) ITALIAN BAKED EGGS IN AVOCADO

Preparation Time: 10 minutes	**Cooking Time:** 15 minutes	**Servings:** 2

✓ One pinch parsley ✓ Two eggs ✓ Two slice bacon	✓ One avocado ✓ 2 tsp chives ✓ One pinch of salt and black pepper	❖ Preheat the oven to 425 degrees. ❖ Break the eggs in a tub, willing to maintain the yolks preserved. ❖ Assemble the avocado halves in the baking bowl, rest them on the side. Slowly spoon one egg yolk in the avocado opening. Keep spooning the white egg into the hole till it is finished. Do the same with leftover egg yolk, egg white, and avocado. Dress with chives, parsley, sea salt, and pepper for each of the avocados. ❖ Gently put the baking dish in the preheated oven and cook for about 15 min well before the eggs are cooked. Sprinkle with bacon over the avocado.

178) SPECIAL GROUND PORK SKILLET

	Cooking Time: 25 Minutes	**Servings:** 4

✓ 1 ½ pounds ground pork ✓ 2 tbsp olive oil ✓ 1 bunch kale, trimmed and roughly chopped ✓ 1 cup onions, sliced ✓ 1/4 tsp black pepper, or more to taste	✓ 1/4 cup tomato puree ✓ 1 bell pepper, chopped ✓ 1 tsp sea salt ✓ 1 cup chicken bone broth ✓ 1/4 cup port wine ✓ 2 cloves garlic, pressed ✓ 1 chili pepper, sliced	❖ Heat tbsp of the olive oil in a cast-iron skillet over a moderately high heat. Now, sauté the onion, garlic, and peppers until they are tender and fragrant; reserve. ❖ Heat the remaining tbsp of olive oil; once hot, cook the ground pork and approximately 5 minutes until no longer pink. ❖ Add in the other ingredients and continue to cook for 15 to 17 minutes or until cooked through. ❖ Storing ❖ Place the ground pork mixture in airtight containers or Ziploc bags; keep in your refrigerator for up to 3 to 4 days. ❖ For freezing, place the ground pork mixture in airtight containers or heavy-duty freezer bags. Freeze up to 2 to 3 months. Defrost in the refrigerator. Bon appétit!

Nutrition: 349 Calories; 13g Fat; 4.4g Carbs; 45.3g Protein; 1.2g Fiber

179) DELICIOUS GREEK STYLE CHEESE PORK

	Cooking Time: 20 Minutes	**Servings:** 6

✓ 1 tbsp sesame oil ✓ 1 ½ pounds pork shoulder, cut into strips ✓ Himalayan salt and freshly ground black pepper, to taste ✓ 1/2 tsp cayenne pepper ✓ 1/2 cup shallots, roughly chopped	✓ 2 bell peppers, sliced ✓ 1/4 cup cream of onion soup ✓ 1/2 tsp Sriracha sauce ✓ 1 tbsp tahini (sesame butter ✓ 1 tbsp soy sauce ✓ 4 ounces gouda cheese, cut into small pieces	❖ Heat he sesame oil in a wok over a moderately high flame. ❖ Stir-fry the pork strips for 3 to 4 minutes or until just browned on all sides. Add in the spices, shallots and bell peppers and continue to cook for a further 4 minutes. ❖ Stir in the cream of onion soup, Sriracha, sesame butter, and soy sauce; continue to cook for to 4 minutes more. ❖ Top with the cheese and continue to cook until the cheese has melted. ❖ Storing ❖ Place your stir-fry in six airtight containers or Ziploc bags; keep in your refrigerator for 3 to 4 days. ❖ For freezing, wrap tightly with heavy-duty aluminum foil or freezer wrap. It will maintain the best quality for 2 to 3 months. Defrost in the refrigerator and reheat in your wok.

Nutrition: 424 Calories; 29.4g Fat; 3. Carbs; 34.2g Protein; 0.6g Fiber

180) SPECIAL PORK IN BLUE CHEESE SAUCE

		Cooking Time: 30 Minutes	Servings: 6

✓ 2 pounds pork center cut loin roast, boneless and cut into 6 pieces ✓ 1 tbsp coconut aminos ✓ 6 ounces blue cheese ✓ 1/3 cup heavy cream ✓ 1/3 cup port wine	✓ 1/3 cup roasted vegetable broth, preferably homemade ✓ 1 tsp dried hot chile flakes ✓ 1 tsp dried rosemary ✓ 1 tbsp lard ✓ 1 shallot, chopped ✓ 2 garlic cloves, chopped ✓ Salt and freshly cracked black peppercorns, to taste	❖ Rub each piece of the pork with salt, black peppercorns, and rosemary. ❖ Melt the lard in a saucepan over a moderately high flame. Sear the pork on all sides about 15 minutes; set aside. ❖ Cook the shallot and garlic until they've softened. Add in port wine to scrape up any brown bits from the bottom. ❖ Reduce the heat to medium-low and add in the remaining ingredients; continue to simmer until the sauce has thickened and reduced. ❖ Storing ❖ Divide the pork and sauce into six portions; place each portion in a separate airtight container or Ziploc bag; keep in your refrigerator for 3 to 4 days. ❖ Freeze the pork and sauce in airtight containers or heavy-duty freezer bags. Freeze up to 4 months. Defrost in the refrigerator. Bon appétit!

Nutrition: 34Calories; 18.9g Fat; 1.9g Carbs; 40.3g Protein; 0.3g Fiber

181) MISSISSIPPI-STYLE PULLED PORK

		Cooking Time: 6 Hours	Servings: 4

✓ 1 ½ pounds pork shoulder ✓ 1 tbsp liquid smoke sauce ✓ 1 tsp chipotle powder	✓ Au Jus gravy seasoning packet ✓ 2 onions, cut into wedges ✓ Kosher salt and freshly ground black pepper, taste	❖ Mix the liquid smoke sauce, chipotle powder, Au Jus gravy seasoning packet, salt and pepper. Rub the spice mixture into the pork on all sides. ❖ Wrap in plastic wrap and let it marinate in your refrigerator for 3 hours. ❖ Prepare your grill for indirect heat. Place the pork butt roast on the grate over a drip pan and top with onions; cover the grill and cook for about 6 hours. ❖ Transfer the pork to a cutting board. Now, shred the meat into bite-sized pieces using two forks. ❖ Storing ❖ Divide the pork between four airtight containers or Ziploc bags; keep in your refrigerator for up to 3 to 5 days. ❖ For freezing, place the pork in airtight containers or heavy-duty freezer bags. Freeze up to 4 months. Defrost in the refrigerator. Bon appétit!

182) SPICY WITH CHEESY TURKEY DIP

		Cooking Time: 25 Minutes	Servings: 4

✓ 1 Fresno chili pepper, deveined and minced ✓ 1 ½ cups Ricotta cheese, creamed, 4% fat, softened ✓ 1/4 cup sour cream ✓ 1 tbsp butter, room temperature ✓ 1 shallot, chopped	✓ 1 tsp garlic, pressed ✓ 1 pound ground turkey ✓ 1/2 cup goat cheese, shredded ✓ Salt and black pepper, to taste ✓ 1 ½ cups Gruyère, shredded	❖ Melt the butter in a frying pan over a moderately high flame. Now, sauté the onion and garlic until they have softened. ❖ Stir in the ground turkey and continue to cook until it is no longer pink. ❖ Transfer the sautéed mixture to a lightly greased baking dish. Add in Ricotta, sour cream, goat cheese, salt, pepper, and chili pepper. ❖ Top with the shredded Gruyère cheese. Bake in the preheated oven at 350 degrees F for about 20 minutes or until hot and bubbly in top. ❖ Storing ❖ Place your dip in an airtight container; keep in your refrigerator for up 3 to 4 days. Enjoy!

183) TURKEY CHORIZO AND BOK CHOY

		Cooking Time: 50 Minutes		Servings: 4

Ingredients	Ingredients	Directions
✓ 4 mild turkey Chorizo, sliced ✓ 1/2 cup full-fat milk ✓ 6 ounces Gruyère cheese, preferably freshly grated ✓ 1 yellow onion, chopped	✓ Coarse salt and ground black pepper, to taste ✓ 1 pound Bok choy, tough stem ends trimmed ✓ 1 cup cream of mushroom soup ✓ 1 tbsp lard, room temperature	❖ Melt the lard in a nonstick skillet over a moderate flame; cook the Chorizo sausage for about 5 minutes, stirring occasionally to ensure even cooking; reserve. ❖ Add in the onion, salt, pepper, Bok choy, and cream of mushroom soup. Continue to cook for 4 minutes longer or until the vegetables have softened. ❖ Spoon the mixture into a lightly oiled casserole dish. Top with the reserved Chorizo. ❖ In a mixing bowl, thoroughly combine the milk and cheese. Pour the cheese mixture over the sausage. ❖ Cover with foil and bake at 36degrees F for about 35 minutes. ❖ Storing ❖ Cut your casserole into four portions. Place each portion in an airtight container; keep in your refrigerator for 3 to 4 days. ❖ For freezing, wrap your portions tightly with heavy-duty aluminum foil or freezer wrap. Freeze up to 1 to 2 months. Defrost in the refrigerator. Enjoy!

184) CLASSIC SPICY CHICKEN BREASTS

		Cooking Time: 30 Minutes		Servings: 6

Ingredients	Ingredients	Directions
✓ 1 ½ pounds chicken breasts ✓ 1 bell pepper, deveined and chopped ✓ 1 leek, chopped ✓ 1 tomato, pureed ✓ 2 tbsp coriander	✓ 2 garlic cloves, minced ✓ 1 tsp cayenne pepper ✓ 1 tsp dry thyme ✓ 1/4 cup coconut aminos ✓ Sea salt and ground black pepper, to taste	❖ Rub each chicken breasts with the garlic, cayenne pepper, thyme, salt and black pepper. Cook the chicken in a saucepan over medium-high heat. ❖ Sear for about 5 minutes until golden brown on all sides. ❖ Fold in the tomato puree and coconut aminos and bring it to a boil. Add in the pepper, leek, and coriander. ❖ Reduce the heat to simmer. Continue to cook, partially covered, for about 20 minutes. ❖ Storing ❖ Place the chicken breasts in airtight containers or Ziploc bags; keep in your refrigerator for 3 to 4 days. ❖ For freezing, place the chicken breasts in airtight containers or heavy-duty freezer bags. It will maintain the best quality for about 4 months. Defrost in the refrigerator. Bon appétit!

185) DELICIOUS SAUCY BOSTON BUTT

		Cooking Time: 1 Hour 20 Minutes		Servings: 8

Ingredients	Ingredients	Directions
✓ 1 tbsp lard, room temperature ✓ 2 pounds Boston butt, cubed ✓ Salt and freshly ground pepper ✓ 1/2 tsp mustard powder ✓ A bunch of spring onions, chopped	✓ 2 garlic cloves, minced ✓ 1/2 tbsp ground cardamom ✓ 2 tomatoes, pureed ✓ 1 bell pepper, deveined and chopped ✓ 1 jalapeno pepper, deveined and finely chopped ✓ 1/2 cup unsweetened coconut milk ✓ 2 cups chicken bone broth	❖ In a wok, melt the lard over moderate heat. Season the pork belly with salt, pepper and mustard powder. ❖ Sear the pork for 8 to 10 minutes, stirring periodically to ensure even cooking; set aside, keeping it warm. ❖ In the same wok, sauté the spring onions, garlic, and cardamom. Spoon the sautéed vegetables along with the reserved pork into the slow cooker. ❖ Add in the remaining ingredients, cover with the lid and cook for 1 hour 10 minutes over low heat. ❖ Divide the pork and vegetables between airtight containers or Ziploc bags; keep in your refrigerator for up to 3 to 5 days. ❖ For freezing, place the pork and vegetables in airtight containers or heavy-duty freezer bags. Freeze up to 4 months. Defrost in the refrigerator. Bon appétit!

186)	SPECIAL OLD-FASHIONED HUNGARIAN GOULASH	
	Cooking Time: 9 Hours 10 Minutes	**Servings: 4**

✓ 1 ½ pounds pork butt, chopped ✓ 1 tsp sweet Hungarian paprika ✓ 2 Hungarian hot peppers, deveined and minced ✓ 1 cup leeks, chopped ✓ 1 ½ tbsp lard ✓ 1 tsp caraway seeds, ground ✓ 4 cups vegetable broth ✓ 2 garlic cloves, crushed ✓ 1 tsp cayenne pepper ✓ 2 cups tomato sauce with herbs	✓ 1 ½ pounds pork butt, chopped ✓ 1 tsp sweet Hungarian paprika ✓ 2 Hungarian hot peppers, deveined and minced ✓ 1 cup leeks, chopped ✓ 1 ½ tbsp lard ✓ 1 tsp caraway seeds, ground ✓ 4 cups vegetable broth ✓ 2 garlic cloves, crushed ✓ 1 tsp cayenne pepper ✓ 2 cups tomato sauce with herbs	❖ Melt the lard in a heavy-bottomed pot over medium-high heat. Sear the pork for 5 to 6 minutes until just browned on all sides; set aside. ❖ Add in the leeks and garlic; continue to cook until they have softened. ❖ Place the reserved pork along with the sautéed mixture in your crock pot. Add in the other ingredients and stir to combine. ❖ Cover with the lid and slow cook for 9 hours on the lowest setting. ❖ Storing ❖ Spoon your goulash into four airtight containers or Ziploc bags; keep in your refrigerator for up to 3 to 4 days. ❖ For freezing, place the goulash in airtight containers. Freeze up to 4 to 6 months. Defrost in the refrigerator. Enjoy!

187)	TYPICAL ITALIAN-STYLE CHEESY PORK LOIN	
	Cooking Time: 25 Minutes	**Servings: 4**

Ingredients:		**Directions:**
✓ 1 pound pork loin, cut into 1-inch-thick pieces ✓ 1 tsp Italian seasoning mix ✓ Salt and pepper, to taste ✓ 1 onion, sliced ✓ 1 tsp fresh garlic, smashed ✓ 2 tbsp black olives, pitted and sliced	✓ 2 tbsp balsamic vinegar ✓ 1/2 cup Romano cheese, grated ✓ 2 tbsp butter, room temperature ✓ 1 tbsp curry paste ✓ 1 cup roasted vegetable broth ✓ 1 tbsp oyster sauce	❖ In a frying pan, melt the butter over a moderately high heat. Once hot, cook the pork until browned on all sides; season with salt and black pepper and set aside. ❖ In the pan drippings, cook the onion and garlic for 4 to 5 minutes or until they've softened. ❖ Add in the Italian seasoning mix, curry paste, and vegetable broth. Continue to cook until the sauce has thickened and reduced slightly or about 10 minutes. Add in the remaining ingredients along with the reserved pork. ❖ Top with cheese and cook for 10 minutes longer or until cooked through. ❖ Storing ❖ Divide the pork loin between four airtight containers; keep in your refrigerator for 3 to 5 days. ❖ For freezing, place the pork loin in airtight containers or heavy-duty freezer bags. Freeze up to 4 to 6 months. Defrost in the refrigerator. Enjoy!

188)	BAKED SPARE RIBS	
	Cooking Time: 3 Hour 40 Minutes	Servings: 6

Ingredients:

- 2 pounds spare ribs
- 1 garlic clove, minced
- 1 tsp dried marjoram
- 1 lime, halved
- Salt and ground black pepper, to taste

Directions:

- Toss all ingredients in a ceramic dish.
- Cover and let it refrigerate for 5 to 6 hours.
- Roast the foil-wrapped ribs in the preheated oven at 275 degrees F degrees for about hours 30 minutes.
- Storing
- Divide the ribs into six portions. Place each portion of ribs in an airtight container; keep in your refrigerator for 3 to days.
- For freezing, place the ribs in airtight containers or heavy-duty freezer bags. Freeze up to 4 to months. Defrost in the refrigerator and reheat in the preheated oven. Bon appétit!

189)	HEALTHY CHICKEN PARMESAN SALAD	
	Cooking Time: 20 Minutes	Servings: 6

- 2 romaine hearts, leaves separated
- Flaky sea salt and ground black pepper, to taste
- 1/4 tsp chili pepper flakes
- 1 tsp dried basil
- 1/4 cup Parmesan, finely grated
- 2 chicken breasts
- 2 Lebanese cucumbers, sliced
- For the dressing:
- 2 large egg yolks
- 1 tsp Dijon mustard
- 1 tbsp fresh lemon juice
- 1/4 cup olive oil
- 2 garlic cloves, minced

Directions:

- In a grilling pan, cook the chicken breast until no longer pink or until a meat thermometer registers 5 degrees F. Slice the chicken into strips.
- Storing
- Place the chicken breasts in airtight containers or Ziploc bags; keep in your refrigerator for to 4 days.
- For freezing, place the chicken breasts in airtight containers or heavy-duty freezer bags. It will maintain the best quality for about months. Defrost in the refrigerator.
- Toss the chicken with the other ingredients. Prepare the dressing by whisking all the ingredients.
- Dress the salad and enjoy! Keep the salad in your refrigerator for 3 to 5 days.

190) CLASSIC TURKEY WINGS WITH GRAVY SAUCE

Cooking Time: 6 Hours	Servings: 6

Ingredients:

- ✓ 2 pounds turkey wings
- ✓ 1/2 tsp cayenne pepper
- ✓ 4 garlic cloves, sliced
- ✓ 1 large onion, chopped
- ✓ Salt and pepper, to taste
- ✓ 1 tsp dried marjoram
- ✓ 1 tbsp butter, room temperature
- ✓ 1 tbsp Dijon mustard
- ✓ For the Gravy:
- ✓ 1 cup double cream
- ✓ Salt and black pepper, to taste
- ✓ 1/2 stick butter
- ✓ 3/4 tsp guar gum

Directions:

- ❖ Rub the turkey wings with the Dijon mustard and tbsp of butter. Preheat a grill pan over medium-high heat.
- ❖ Sear the turkey wings for 10 minutes on all sides.
- ❖ Transfer the turkey to your Crock pot; add in the garlic, onion, salt, pepper, marjoram, and cayenne pepper. Cover and cook on low setting for 6 hours.
- ❖ Melt 1/2 stick of the butter in a frying pan. Add in the cream and whisk until cooked through.
- ❖ Next, stir in the guar gum, salt, and black pepper along with cooking juices. Let it cook until the sauce has reduced by half.
- ❖ Storing
- ❖ Wrap the turkey wings in foil before packing them into airtight containers; keep in your refrigerator for up to 3 to 4 days.
- ❖ For freezing, place the turkey wings in airtight containers or heavy-duty freezer bags. Freeze up to 2 to 3 months. Defrost in the refrigerator.
- ❖ Keep your gravy in refrigerator for up to 2 days.

191) AUTHENTIC PORK CHOPS WITH HERBS

Cooking Time: 20 Minutes	Servings: 4

Ingredients:

- ✓ 1 tbsp butter
- ✓ 1 pound pork chops
- ✓ 2 rosemary sprigs, minced
- ✓ 1 tsp dried marjoram
- ✓ 1 tsp dried parsley
- ✓ A bunch of spring onions, roughly chopped
- ✓ 1 thyme sprig, minced
- ✓ 1/2 tsp granulated garlic
- ✓ 1/2 tsp paprika, crushed
- ✓ Coarse salt and ground black pepper, to taste

- ❖ Season the pork chops with the granulated garlic, paprika, salt, and black pepper.
- ❖ Melt the butter in a frying pan over a moderate flame. Cook the pork chops for 6 to 8 minutes, turning them occasionally to ensure even cooking.
- ❖ Add in the remaining ingredients and cook an additional 4 minutes.
- ❖ Storing
- ❖ Divide the pork chops into four portions; place each portion in a separate airtight container or Ziploc bag; keep in your refrigerator for 3 to 4 days.
- ❖ Freeze the pork chops in airtight containers or heavy-duty freezer bags. Freeze up to 4 months. Defrost in the refrigerator. Bon appétit!

192) PEPPERS STUFFED WITH CHOPPED PORK ORIGINAL

Cooking Time: 40 Minutes	Servings: 4

Ingredients:

- ✓ 6 bell peppers, deveined
- ✓ 1 tbsp vegetable oil
- ✓ 1 shallot, chopped
- ✓ 1 garlic clove, minced
- ✓ 1/2 pound ground pork
- ✓ 1/3 pound ground veal
- ✓ 1 ripe tomato, chopped
- ✓ 1/2 tsp mustard seeds
- ✓ Sea salt and ground black pepper, to taste

- ❖ Parboil the peppers for 5 minutes.
- ❖ Heat the vegetable oil in a frying pan that is preheated over a moderate heat. Cook the shallot and garlic for 3 to 4 minutes until they've softened.
- ❖ Stir in the ground meat and cook, breaking apart with a fork, for about 6 minutes. Add the chopped tomatoes, mustard seeds, salt, and pepper.
- ❖ Continue to cook for 5 minutes or until heated through. Divide the filling between the peppers and transfer them to a baking pan.
- ❖ Bake in the preheated oven at 36degrees F approximately 25 minutes.
- ❖ Storing
- ❖ Place the peppers in airtight containers or Ziploc bags; keep in your refrigerator for up to 3 to 4 days.
- ❖ For freezing, place the peppers in airtight containers or heavy-duty freezer bags. Freeze up to 2 to 3 months. Defrost in the refrigerator. Bon appétit!

Nutrition: 2 Calories; 20.5g Fat; 8.2g Carbs; 18.2g Protein; 1.5g Fiber

193) GRILL-STYLE CHICKEN SALAD WITH AVOCADO

	Cooking Time: 20 Minutes	Servings: 4

Ingredients:

- ✓ 1/3 cup olive oil
- ✓ 2 chicken breasts
- ✓ Sea salt and crushed red pepper flakes
- ✓ 2 egg yolks
- ✓ 1 tbsp fresh lemon juice
- ✓ 1/2 tsp celery seeds
- ✓ 1 tbsp coconut aminos
- ✓ 1 large-sized avocado, pitted and sliced

Directions:

- ❖ Grill the chicken breasts for about 4 minutes per side. Season with salt and pepper, to taste.
- ❖ Slice the grilled chicken into bite-sized strips.
- ❖ To make the dressing, whisk the egg yolks, lemon juice, celery seeds, olive oil and coconut aminos in a measuring cup.
- ❖ Storing
- ❖ Place the chicken breasts in airtight containers or Ziploc bags; keep in your refrigerator for 3 to 4 days.
- ❖ For freezing, place the chicken breasts in airtight containers or heavy-duty freezer bags. It will maintain the best quality for about 4 months. Defrost in the refrigerator.
- ❖ Store dressing in your refrigerator for 3 to 4 days. Dress the salad and garnish with fresh avocado. Bon appétit!

194) EASY TO COOK RIBS

	Cooking Time: 8 Hours	Servings: 4

- ✓ 1 pound baby back ribs
- ✓ 4 tbsp coconut aminos
- ✓ 1/4 cup dry red wine
- ✓ 1/2 tsp cayenne pepper
- ✓ 1 garlic clove, crushed
- ✓ 1 tsp Italian herb mix
- ✓ 1 tbsp butter
- ✓ 1 tsp Serrano pepper, minced
- ✓ 1 Italian pepper, thinly sliced
- ✓ 1 tsp grated lemon zest

- ❖ Butter the sides and bottom of your Crock pot. Place the pork and peppers on the bottom.
- ❖ Add in the remaining ingredients.
- ❖ Slow cook for 9 hours on Low heat setting.
- ❖ Storing
- ❖ Divide the baby back ribs into four portions. Place each portion of the ribs along with the peppers in an airtight container; keep in your refrigerator for 3 days.
- ❖ For freezing, place the ribs in airtight containers or heavy-duty freezer bags. Freeze up to 4 to months. Defrost in the refrigerator. Reheat in your oven at 250 degrees F until heated through.

195) CLASSIC BRIE-STUFFED MEATBALLS

	Cooking Time: 25 Minutes	Servings: 5

- ✓ 2 eggs, beaten
- ✓ 1 pound ground pork
- ✓ 1/3 cup double cream
- ✓ 1 tbsp fresh parsley
- ✓ Kosher salt and ground black pepper
- ✓ 1 tsp dried rosemary
- ✓ 10 (1-inch cubes of brie cheese
- ✓ 2 tbsp scallions, minced
- ✓ 2 cloves garlic, minced

- ❖ Mix all ingredients, except for the brie cheese, until everything is well incorporated.
- ❖ Roll the mixture into 10 patties; place a piece of cheese in the center of each patty and roll into a ball.
- ❖ Roast in the preheated oven at 0 degrees F for about 20 minutes.
- ❖ Storing
- ❖ Place the meatballs in airtight containers or Ziploc bags; keep in your refrigerator for up to 3 to 4 days.
- ❖ Freeze the meatballs in airtight containers or heavy-duty freezer bags. Freeze up to 3 to 4 months. To defrost, slowly reheat in a saucepan. Bon appétit!

Nutrition: 302 Calories; 13g Fat; 1.9g Carbs; 33.4g Protein; 0.3g Fiber

196) ORANGE WITH WHOLE COUSCOUS SCENTED WITH CINNAMON

Cooking Time: 10 Minutes	Servings: 4

Ingredients:

- ✓ 2 tsp olive oil
- ✓ ¼ cup minced shallot
- ✓ ½ cup freshly squeezed orange juice (from 2 oranges)
- ✓ ½ cup water
- ✓ ⅛ tsp ground cinnamon
- ✓ ¼ tsp kosher salt
- ✓ 1 cup whole-wheat couscous

Directions:

- ❖ Heat the oil in a saucepan over medium heat. Once the oil is shimmering, add the shallot and cook for 2 minutes, stirring frequently. Add the orange juice, water, cinnamon, and salt, and bring to a boil.
- ❖ Once the liquid is boiling, add the couscous, cover the pan, and turn off the heat. Leave the couscous covered for 5 minutes. When the couscous is done, fluff with a fork.
- ❖ Place ¾ cup of couscous in each of 4 containers.
- ❖ STORAGE: Store covered containers in the refrigerator for up to 5 days. Freeze for up to 2 months.

Nutrition: Total calories: 21 Total fat: 4g; Saturated fat: <1g; Sodium: 147mg; Carbohydrates: 41g; Fiber: 5g; Protein: 8g

197) CHUNKY ROASTED CHERRY TOMATO WITH BASIL SAUCE

Cooking Time: 40 Minutes	Servings: 1⅓ Cups

Ingredients:

- ✓ 2 pints cherry tomatoes (20 ounces total)
- ✓ 2 tsp olive oil, plus 3 tbsp
- ✓ ¼ tsp kosher salt
- ✓ ½ tsp chopped garlic
- ✓ ¼ cup fresh basil leaves

Directions:

- ❖ Preheat the oven to 350°F. Line a sheet pan with a silicone baking mat or parchment paper.
- ❖ Place the tomatoes on the lined sheet pan and toss with tsp of oil. Roast for 40 minutes, shaking the pan halfway through.
- ❖ While the tomatoes are still warm, place them in a medium mixing bowl and add the salt, the garlic, and the remaining tbsp of oil. Mash the tomatoes with the back of a fork. Stir in the fresh basil.
- ❖ Scoop the sauce into a container and refrigerate.
- ❖ STORAGE: Store the covered container in the refrigerator for up to days.

Nutrition: (⅓ cup): Total calories: 141; Total fat: 13g; Saturated fat: 2g; Sodium: 158mg; Carbohydrates: 7g; Fiber: 2g; Protein: 1g

198) PESTO OF CELERY HEARTS, BASIL AND ALMONDS

Cooking Time: 10 Minutes	Servings: 1 Cup

Ingredients:

- ✓ ½ cup raw, unsalted almonds
- ✓ 3 cups fresh basil leaves, (about 1½ ounces)
- ✓ ½ cup chopped celery hearts with leaves
- ✓ ¼ tsp kosher salt
- ✓ 1 tbsp freshly squeezed lemon juice
- ✓ ¼ cup olive oil
- ✓ 3 tbsp water

Directions:

- ❖ Place the almonds in the bowl of a food processor and process until they look like coarse sand.
- ❖ Add the basil, celery hearts, salt, lemon juice, oil and water and process until smooth. The sauce will be somewhat thick. If you would like a thinner sauce, add more water, oil, or lemon juice, depending on your taste preference.
- ❖ Scoop the pesto into a container and refrigerate.
- ❖ STORAGE: Store the covered container in the refrigerator for up to 2 weeks. Pesto may be frozen for up to 6 months.

Nutrition: (¼ cup): Total calories: 231; Total fat: 22g; Saturated fat: 3g; Sodium: 178mg; Carbohydrates: 6g; Fiber: 3g; Protein: 4g

199) SAUTÉED KALE AND GARLIC WITH LEMON

	Cooking Time: 7 Minutes	Servings: 4

Ingredients:

- ✓ 1 tbsp olive oil
- ✓ 3 bunches kale, stemmed and roughly chopped
- ✓ 2 tsp chopped garlic
- ✓ ¼ tsp kosher salt
- ✓ 1 tbsp freshly squeezed lemon juice

Directions:

- ❖ Heat the oil in a -inch skillet over medium-high heat. Once the oil is shimmering, add as much kale as will fit in the pan. You will probably only fit half the leaves into the pan at first. Mix the kale with tongs so that the leaves are coated with oil and start to wilt. As the kale wilts, keep adding more of the raw kale, continuing to use tongs to mix. Once all the kale is in the pan, add the garlic and salt and continue to cook until the kale is tender. Total cooking time from start to finish should be about 7 minutes.
- ❖ Mix the lemon juice into the kale. Add additional salt and/or lemon juice if necessary. Place 1 cup of kale in each of 4 containers and refrigerate.
- ❖ STORAGE: Store covered containers in the refrigerator for up to 5 days

Nutrition: Total calories: 8 Total fat: 1g; Saturated fat: <1g; Sodium: 214mg; Carbohydrates: 17g; Fiber: 6g; Protein: 6g

200) CREAMY POLENTA AND CHIVES WITH PARMESAN

	Cooking Time: 15 Minutes	Servings: 5

Ingredients:

- ✓ 1 tsp olive oil
- ✓ ¼ cup minced shallot
- ✓ ½ cup white wine
- ✓ 3¼ cups water
- ✓ ¾ cup cornmeal
- ✓ 3 tbsp grated Parmesan cheese
- ✓ ½ tsp kosher salt
- ✓ ¼ cup chopped chives

Directions:

- ❖ Heat the oil in a saucepan over medium heat. Once the oil is shimmering, add the shallot and sauté for 2 minutes. Add the wine and water and bring to a boil.
- ❖ Pour the cornmeal in a thin, even stream into the liquid, stirring continuously until the mixture starts to thicken.
- ❖ Reduce the heat to low and continue to cook for 10 to 12 minutes, whisking every 1 to 2 minutes.
- ❖ Turn the heat off and stir in the cheese, salt, and chives. Cool.
- ❖ Place about ¾ cup of polenta in each of containers.
- ❖ STORAGE: Store covered containers in the refrigerator for up to 5 days.

Nutrition: Total calories: 110; Total fat: 3g; Saturated fat: 1g; Sodium: 29g; Carbohydrates: 16g; Fiber: 1g; Protein: 3g

201) SPECIAL MOCHA-NUT STUFFED DATES

	Cooking Time: 10 Minutes	Servings: 5

Ingredients:

- ✓ 2 tbsp creamy, unsweetened, unsalted almond butter
- ✓ 1 tsp unsweetened cocoa powder
- ✓ 3 tbsp walnut pieces
- ✓ 2 tbsp water
- ✓ ¼ tsp honey
- ✓ ¾ tsp instant espresso powder
- ✓ 10 Medjool dates, pitted

Directions:

- ❖ In a small bowl, combine the almond butter, cocoa powder, and walnut pieces.
- ❖ Place the water in a small microwaveable mug and heat on high for 30 seconds. Add the honey and espresso powder to the water and stir to dissolve.
- ❖ Add the espresso water to the cocoa bowl and combine thoroughly until a creamy, thick paste forms.
- ❖ Stuff each pitted date with 1 tsp of mocha filling.
- ❖ Place 2 dates in each of small containers.
- ❖ STORAGE: Store covered containers in the refrigerator for up to 5 days.

Nutrition: Total calories: 205; Total fat: ; Saturated fat: 1g; Sodium: 1mg; Carbohydrates: 39g; Fiber: 4g; Protein: 3g

202)	SPECIAL EGGPLANT DIP ROAST (BABA GHANOUSH)	
	Cooking Time: 45 Minutes	**Servings:** 2 Cups

Ingredients:

- ✓ 2 eggplants (close to 1 pound each)
- ✓ 1 tsp chopped garlic
- ✓ 3 tbsp unsalted tahini
- ✓ ¼ cup freshly squeezed lemon juice
- ✓ 1 tbsp olive oil
- ✓ ½ tsp kosher salt

Directions:

- ❖ Preheat the oven to 450°F and line a sheet pan with a silicone baking mat or parchment paper.
- ❖ Prick the eggplants in many places with a fork, place on the sheet pan, and roast in the oven until extremely soft, about 45 minutes. The eggplants should look like they are deflating.
- ❖ When the eggplants are cool, cut them open and scoop the flesh into a large bowl. You may need to use your hands to pull the flesh away from the skin. Discard the skin. Mash the flesh very well with a fork.
- ❖ Add the garlic, tahini, lemon juice, oil, and salt. Taste and adjust the seasoning with additional lemon juice, salt, or tahini if needed.
- ❖ Scoop the dip into a container and refrigerate.
- ❖ STORAGE: Store the covered container in the refrigerator for up to 5 days.

Nutrition: (¼ cup): Total calories: 8 Total fat: 5g; Saturated fat: 1g; Sodium: 156mg; Carbohydrates: 10g; Fiber: 4g; Protein: 2g

203)	DELICIOUS HONEY-LEMON VINAIGRETTE	
	Cooking Time: 5 Minutes	**Servings:** ½ Cup

- ✓ ¼ cup freshly squeezed lemon juice
- ✓ 1 tsp honey
- ✓ 2 tsp Dijon mustard
- ✓ ⅛ tsp kosher salt
- ✓ ¼ cup olive oil

- ❖ Place the lemon juice, honey, mustard, and salt in a small bowl and whisk to combine.
- ❖ Whisk in the oil, pouring it into the bowl in a thin steam.
- ❖ Pour the vinaigrette into a container and refrigerate.
- ❖ STORAGE: Store the covered container in the refrigerator for up to 2 weeks. Allow the vinaigrette to come to room temperature and shake before serving.

Nutrition: (2 tbsp): Total calories: 131; Total fat: 14g; Saturated fat: 2g; Sodium: 133mg; Carbohydrates: 3g; Fiber: <1g; Protein: <1g

204)	SPANISH-STYLE ROMESCO SAUCE	
	Cooking Time: 10 Minutes	**Servings:** 1⅔ Cups

- ✓ ½ cup raw, unsalted almonds
- ✓ 4 medium garlic cloves (do not peel)
- ✓ 1 (12-ounce) jar of roasted red peppers, drained
- ✓ ½ cup canned diced fire-roasted tomatoes, drained
- ✓ 1 tsp smoked paprika
- ✓ ½ tsp kosher salt
- ✓ Pinch cayenne pepper
- ✓ 2 tsp red wine vinegar
- ✓ 2 tbsp olive oil

- ❖ Preheat the oven to 350°F.
- ❖ Place the almonds and garlic cloves on a sheet pan and toast in the oven for 10 minutes. Remove from the oven and peel the garlic when cool enough to handle.
- ❖ Place the almonds in the bowl of a food processor. Process the almonds until they resemble coarse sand, to 45 seconds. Add the garlic, peppers, tomatoes, paprika, salt, and cayenne. Blend until smooth.
- ❖ Once the mixture is smooth, add the vinegar and oil and blend until well combined. Taste and add more vinegar or salt if needed.
- ❖ Scoop the romesco sauce into a container and refrigerate.
- ❖ STORAGE: Store the covered container in the refrigerator for up to 7 days.

Nutrition: (⅓ cup): Total calories: 158; Total fat: 13g; Saturated fat: 1g; Sodium: 292mg; Carbohydrates: 10g; Fiber: 3g; Protein: 4g

205) MASCARPONE WITH CARDAMOM AND STRAWBERRIES

Cooking Time: 10 Minutes	**Servings: 4**

Ingredients	Ingredients	Instructions
✓ 1 (8-ounce) container mascarpone cheese ✓ 2 tsp honey	✓ ¼ tsp ground cardamom ✓ 2 tbsp milk ✓ 1 pound strawberries (should be 24 strawberries in the pack)	❖ Combine the mascarpone, honey, cardamom, and milk in a medium mixing bowl. ❖ Mix the ingredients with a spoon until super creamy, about 30 seconds. ❖ Place 6 strawberries and 2 tbsp of the mascarpone mixture in each of 4 containers. ❖ STORAGE: Store covered containers in the refrigerator for up to 5 days.

206) SWEET AND SPICY GREEN PUMPKIN SEEDS

Cooking Time: 15 Minutes	**Servings: 2 Cups**

Ingredients	Ingredients	Instructions
✓ 2 cups raw green pumpkin seeds (pepitas) ✓ 1 egg white, beaten until frothy ✓ 3 tbsp honey	✓ 1 tbsp chili powder ✓ ¼ tsp cayenne pepper ✓ 1 tsp ground cinnamon ✓ ¼ tsp kosher salt	❖ Preheat the oven to 350°F. Line a sheet pan with a silicone baking mat or parchment paper. ❖ In a medium bowl, mix all the ingredients until the seeds are well coated. Place on the lined sheet pan in a single, even layer. ❖ Bake for 15 minutes. Cool the seeds on the sheet pan, then peel clusters from the baking mat and break apart into small pieces. ❖ Place ¼ cup of seeds in each of 8 small containers or resealable sandwich bags.

207) Shrimp and Penne

Cooking Time: 35 Minutes	**Servings: 8**

Ingredients	Ingredients	Instructions
✓ Penne pasta (16 oz. pkg.) ✓ Salt (.25 tsp.) ✓ Olive oil (2 tbsp.) ✓ Diced tomatoes (2 - 14.5 oz. cans)	✓ Garlic (1 tbsp.) ✓ Red onion (.25 cup) ✓ White wine (.25 cup) ✓ Shrimp (1 lb.) ✓ Grated parmesan cheese (1 cup)	❖ Dice the red onion and garlic. Peel and devein the shrimp. ❖ Add salt to a large soup pot of water and set it on the stovetop to boil. Add the pasta and cook for nine to ten minutes. Drain it thoroughly in a colander. ❖ Empty oil into a skillet. Warm it using the medium temperature setting. ❖ Toss in the garlic and onion to sauté until they're tender. ❖ Pour in the tomatoes and wine. Continue cooking for about ten minutes, stirring occasionally. ❖ Fold in the shrimp and continue cooking for about five minutes or until it's opaque. ❖ Combine the pasta and shrimp and top it off with the cheese to serve.

208)	CHICKPEA SALAD WITH BRUSSELS SPROUTS	
	Cooking Time: 10 Minutes	Servings: 4

✓ 1 cup roasted chickpeas. To give the dish a saltier taste, you can add sea salt. ✓ 4 cups kale, chopped	✓ 9 ounces Brussels sprouts, shredded ✓ 1 avocado, peeled, pitted, and cut	❖ Divide the kale and Brussels sprouts into four bowls. ❖ Add the chickpeas and the avocado. ❖ You can add a little sea salt and/or pepper to taste. Another tip for more taste is to drizzle a little Vinaigrette dressing or your favorite homemade Italian-Style dressing.

Nutrition: calories: 337, fats: 20 grams, carbohydrates: 30 grams, protein: 12 grams.

209)	MEAT LOAF	
	Cooking Time: 1 Hour 15 Minutes	Servings: 12

✓ 1 garlic clove, minced ✓ ½ tsp dried thyme, crushed ✓ ½ pound grass-fed lean ground beef ✓ 1 organic egg, beaten ✓ Salt and black pepper, to taste ✓ ¼ cup onions, chopped	✓ 1/8 cup sugar-free ketchup ✓ 2 cups mozzarella cheese, freshly grated ✓ ¼ cup green bell pepper, seeded and chopped ✓ ½ cup cheddar cheese, grated ✓ 1 cup fresh spinach, chopped	❖ Preheat the oven to 350 degrees F and grease a baking dish. ❖ Put all the ingredients in a bowl except spinach and cheese and mix well. ❖ Arrange the meat over a wax paper and top with spinach and cheese. ❖ Roll the paper around the mixture to form a meatloaf. ❖ Remove the wax paper and transfer the meat loaf in the baking dish. ❖ Put it in the oven and bake for about 1 hour. ❖ Dish out and serve hot. ❖ Meal Prep Tip: Let the meat loafs cool for about 10 minutes to bring them to room temperature before serving.

210)	COUSCOUS WITH PEPPERONCINI AND TUNA	
	Cooking Time: 20 Minutes	Servings: 4

✓ The Couscous: ✓ Chicken broth or water (1 cup) ✓ Couscous (1.25 cups) ✓ Kosher salt (.75 tsp.) ✓ The Accompaniments: ✓ Cherry tomatoes (1 pint - halved)	✓ Sliced pepperoncini(.5 cup) ✓ Chopped fresh parsley (.33 cup) ✓ Capers (.25 cup) ✓ Olive oil (for serving) ✓ Black pepper & kosher salt (as desired) ✓ Lemon (1 quartered) ✓ Oil-pack tuna (2.5oz cans)	❖ Make the couscous in a small saucepan using water or broth. Prepare it using the medium heat temperature setting. Let it sit for about ten minutes. ❖ Toss the tomatoes, tuna, capers, parsley, and pepperoncini into a mixing bowl. ❖ Fluff the couscous when done and dust using the pepper and salt. Spritz it using the oil and serve with the tuna mix and a lemon wedge.

211) TILAPIA WITH AVOCADO AND RED ONION

	Cooking Time: 15 Minutes	Servings: 4

Ingredients:

- ✓ Olive oil (1 tbsp.)
- ✓ Sea salt (.25 tsp.)
- ✓ Fresh orange juice (1 tbsp.)
- ✓ Tilapia fillets (four 4 oz. - more rectangular than square)
- ✓ Red onion (.25 cup)
- ✓ Sliced avocado (1)
- ✓ Also Needed: 9-inch pie plate

Directions:

- ❖ Combine the salt, juice, and oil to add into the pie dish. Work with one fillet at a time. Place it in the dish and turn to coat all sides.
- ❖ Arrange the fillets in a wagon wheel-shaped formation. (Each of the fillets should be in the center of the dish with the other end draped over the edge.
- ❖ Place a tbsp of the onion on top of each of the fillets and fold the end into the center. Cover the dish with plastic wrap, leaving one corner open to vent the steam.
- ❖ Place in the microwave using the high heat setting for three minutes. It's done when the center can be easily flaked.
- ❖ Top the fillets off with avocado and serve.

Nutrition: Calories: 200;Protein: 22 grams;Fat: 11 grams

212) BAKED SALMON AND DILL

	Cooking Time: 15 Minutes	Servings: 4

- ✓ Salmon fillets (4- 6 oz. portions - 1-inch thickness)
- ✓ Kosher salt (.5 tsp.)
- ✓ Finely chopped fresh dill (1.5 tbsp.)
- ✓ Black pepper (.125 tsp.)
- ✓ Lemon wedges (4)

- ❖ Warm the oven in advance to reach 350° Fahrenheit.
- ❖ Lightly grease a baking sheet with a misting of cooking oil spray and add the fish. Lightly spritz the fish with the spray along with a shake of salt, pepper, and dill.
- ❖ Bake it until the fish is easily flaked (10 min..)
- ❖ Serve with lemon wedges.

213) STEAK WITH VEGETABLES

	Cooking Time: 15 Minutes	Servings: 6

- ✓ 2 lbs baby red potatoes
- ✓ 16 oz broccoli florets
- ✓ 2 tbsp olive oil
- ✓ 3 cloves garlic, minced
- ✓ 1 tsp dried thyme
- ✓ Kosher salt, to taste
- ✓ Freshly ground black pepper, to taste
- ✓ 2 lbs (1-inch-thick) top sirloin steak, patted dry

- ❖ Preheat oven to broil
- ❖ Lightly oil a baking sheet or coat with nonstick spray
- ❖ In a large pot over high heat, boil salted water, cook the potatoes until parboiled for 12-15 minutes, drain well
- ❖ Place the potatoes and broccoli in a single layer onto the prepared baking sheet
- ❖ Add the olive oil, garlic and thyme, season with salt and pepper, to taste and then gently toss to combine
- ❖ Season the steaks with salt and pepper, to taste, and add to the baking sheet in a single layer
- ❖ Place it into oven and broil until the steak is browned and charred at the edges, about 4-5 minutes per side for medium-rare, or until the desired doneness
- ❖ Distribute the steak and veggies among the containers. Store in the fridge for up to 3 days
- ❖ To Serve: Reheat in the microwave for 1-2 minutes. Top with garlic butter and enjoy

214)	Fattoush special salad	
	Cooking Time: 10 Minutes	**Servings: 4**

✓ 2 loaves pita bread ✓ 3 tbsp extra virgin olive oil ✓ ½ tsp of sumac ✓ salt ✓ pepper ✓ 1 heart romaine lettuce, chopped ✓ 1 English cucumber, chopped ✓ 5 Roma tomatoes, chopped ✓ 5 green onions, chopped	✓ 5 radishes, stems removed, thinly sliced ✓ 2 cups fresh parsley leaves, stems removed, chopped ✓ 1 cup fresh mint leaves, chopped ✓ lime juice, 1½ limes ✓ 1/3 bottle extra virgin olive oil ✓ salt ✓ pepper ✓ 1 tsp ground sumac ✓ ¼ tsp ground cinnamon ✓ scant ¼ tsp ground allspice	❖ Toast pita bread until crisp but not browned. ❖ Heat 3 tbsp of olive oil in a large pan over medium heat. ❖ Break the toasted pita into pieces and add them to the oil. ❖ Fry pita bread until browned, making sure to toss them from time to time. ❖ Add salt, ½ a tsp of sumac, and pepper. ❖ Remove the pita from the heat and place on a paper towel to drain. ❖ In a large mixing bowl, combine lettuce, tomatoes, cucumber, green onions, parsley, and radish. ❖ Before serving, make the lime vinaigrette by mixing all Ingredients: listed above under vinaigrette in a separate bowl. ❖ Pour the vinaigrette over the Ingredients: in the other bowl and gently toss. ❖ Add pita chips on top and the remaining sumac. ❖ Give it a final toss and enjoy

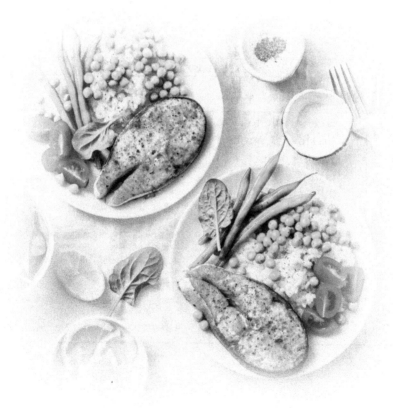

96

215) ROASTED CHICKEN

	Cooking Time: 1 – 1 ½ Hour	Servings: 6

Ingredients:

- ✓ fresh orange juice, 1 large orange
- ✓ ¼ cup Dijon mustard
- ✓ ¼ cup olive oil
- ✓ 4 tsp dried Greek oregano
- ✓ salt
- ✓ ground black pepper
- ✓ 12 potatoes, peeled and cubed
- ✓ 5 garlic cloves, minced
- ✓ 1 whole chicken

Directions:

- ❖ Preheat oven to 375 degrees F.
- ❖ Take a bowl and whisk in orange juice, Greek oregano, Dijon mustard, salt, and pepper. Mix well.
- ❖ Add potatoes to the bowl and coat them thoroughly.
- ❖ Transfer the potatoes to a large baking dish, leaving remaining juice in a bowl.
- ❖ Stuff the garlic cloves into your chicken (under the skin).
- ❖ Place the chicken into the bowl with the remaining juice and coat it thoroughly.
- ❖ Transfer chicken to the baking dish, placing it on top of the potatoes.
- ❖ Pour any extra juice on top of chicken and potatoes.
- ❖ Bake uncovered until the thickest part of the chicken registers 160 degrees F, and the juices run clear, anywhere from 60 – minutes.
- ❖ Remove the chicken and cover it with doubled aluminum foil.
- ❖ Allow it to rest for 10 minutes.
- ❖ Slice, spread over containers and enjoy!

216) Special Pomegranate Vinaigrette

	Cooking Time: 5 Minutes	Servings: ½ Cup

Ingredients:

- ✓ ⅓ cup pomegranate juice
- ✓ 1 tsp Dijon mustard
- ✓ 1 tbsp apple cider vinegar
- ✓ ½ tsp dried mint
- ✓ 2 tbsp plus 2 tsp olive oil

Directions:

- ❖ Place the pomegranate juice, mustard, vinegar, and mint in a small bowl and whisk to combine.
- ❖ Whisk in the oil, pouring it into the bowl in a thin steam.
- ❖ Pour the vinaigrette into a container and refrigerate.
- ❖ STORAGE: Store the covered container in the refrigerator for up to 2 weeks. Bring the vinaigrette to room temperature and shake before serving.

Nutrition: (2 tbsp): Total calories: 94; Total fat: 10g; Saturated fat: 2g; Sodium: 30mg; Carbohydrates: 3g; Fiber: 0g; Protein: 0g

217) GREEN OLIVE WITH SPINACH TAPENADE

	Cooking Time: 20 Minutes	Servings: 1½ Cups

Ingredients:

- ✓ 1 cup pimento-stuffed green olives, drained
- ✓ 3 packed cups baby spinach
- ✓ 1 tsp chopped garlic
- ✓ ½ tsp dried oregano
- ✓ ⅓ cup packed fresh basil
- ✓ 2 tbsp olive oil
- ✓ 2 tsp red wine vinegar

Directions:

- ❖ Place all the ingredients in the bowl of a food processor and pulse until the mixture looks finely chopped but not puréed.
- ❖ Scoop the tapenade into a container and refrigerate.
- ❖ STORAGE: Store the covered container in the refrigerator for up to 5 days.

Nutrition: (¼ cup): Total calories: 80; Total fat: 8g; Saturated fat: 1g; Sodium: 6mg; Carbohydrates: 1g; Fiber: 1g; Protein: 1g

218) BULGUR PILAF AND ALMONDS

Cooking Time: 20 Minutes	Servings: 4

Ingredients:

- ✓ ²⁄₃ cup uncooked bulgur
- ✓ 1¹⁄₃ cups water
- ✓ ¼ cup sliced almonds
- ✓ 1 cup small diced red bell pepper
- ✓ ¹⁄₃ cup chopped fresh cilantro
- ✓ 1 tbsp olive oil
- ✓ ¼ tsp salt

Directions:

- ❖ Place the bulgur and water in a saucepan and bring the water to a boil. Once the water is at a boil, cover the pot with a lid and turn off the heat. Let the covered pot stand for 20 minutes.
- ❖ Transfer the cooked bulgur to a large mixing bowl and add the almonds, peppers, cilantro, oil, and salt. Stir to combine.
- ❖ Place about 1 cup of bulgur in each of 4 containers.
- ❖ STORAGE: Store covered containers in the refrigerator for up to 5 days. Bulgur can be either reheated or eaten at room temperature.

219) EASY SPANISH GARLIC YOGURT SAUCE

Cooking Time: 5 Minutes	Servings: 1 Cup

Ingredients:

- ✓ 1 cup low-fat (2%) plain Greek yogurt
- ✓ ½ tsp garlic powder
- ✓ 1 tbsp freshly squeezed lemon juice
- ✓ 1 tbsp olive oil
- ✓ ¼ tsp kosher salt

Directions:

- ❖ Mix all the ingredients in a medium bowl until well combined.
- ❖ Spoon the yogurt sauce into a container and refrigerate.
- ❖ STORAGE: Store the covered container in the refrigerator for up to 7 days

220) Chicken with balsamic vinegar and vegetables skewers

Cooking Time: 25 Minutes	Servings: 4

Ingredients:

- ✓ 1 pound boneless, skinless chicken breasts, cut into 1-inch cubes
- ✓ ¹⁄₃ cup balsamic vinegar
- ✓ 4 tbsp olive oil, divided
- ✓ 4 tsp dried Italian herbs, divided
- ✓ 2 tsp garlic powder, divided
- ✓ 2 tsp onion powder, divided
- ✓ 8 ounces whole button or cremini mushrooms, stems removed
- ✓ 1 large red bell pepper, cut into 1-inch squares
- ✓ 1 small red onion, quartered and layers pulled apart
- ✓ 1 large zucchini, sliced into ½-inch rounds
- ✓ ¾ tsp kosher salt
- ✓ 8 (11¾-inch) wooden or metal skewers, soaked in water for at least 1 hour if wooden

Directions:

- ❖ Preheat the oven to 450°F. Line a sheet pan with aluminum foil.
- ❖ Place the chicken in a gallon-size resealable bag along with the balsamic vinegar, tbsp of oil, 2 tsp of Italian herbs, 1 tsp of garlic powder, and 1 tsp of onion powder. Seal the bag and make sure all the pieces of chicken are coated with marinade.
- ❖ In a second resealable bag, place the mushrooms, bell pepper, onion, and zucchini and the remaining 2 tbsp of oil, 2 tsp of Italian herbs, 1 tsp of garlic powder, and 1 tsp of onion powder. Seal the bag and shake to make sure the veggies are coated.
- ❖ Refrigerate both bags and marinate for at least 2 hours.
- ❖ Thread the chicken and veggies on 8 skewers, alternating both chicken and veggies on each skewer. Place 6 skewers vertically in the center of the pan, 1 horizontally at the top, and 1 at the bottom. Sprinkle half the salt over the skewers, then flip over and sprinkle the skewers with the remaining salt.
- ❖ Bake for 15 minutes, carefully flip the skewers, then bake for another 10 minutes. Cool.
- ❖ If you have containers long enough to fit the skewers, place 2 skewers directly in each of 4 containers. If not, break the skewers in half or slide the meat and veggies off the skewers.
- ❖ STORAGE: Store covered containers in the refrigerator for up to 5 days.

Nutrition: Total calories: 224; Total fat: 10g; Saturated fat: 2g; Sodium: 631mg; Carbohydrates: 11g; Fiber: 3g; Protein: 27g

221) PESTO CHICKEN WITH TOMATO ZOODLES

	Cooking Time: 15 Minutes	Servings: 4

Ingredients	Ingredients	Instructions
✓ 3 Zucchini, inspiralized ✓ 2 boneless skinless chicken breasts ✓ 1 1/2 cup cherry tomatoes ✓ 2 tsp olive oil	✓ 1/2 tsp salt ✓ Store brought Pesto or Homemade Basil Pesto ✓ Salt, to taste ✓ Pepper, to taste	❖ Preheat grill to medium high heat ❖ Season both sides of the chicken with salt and pepper ❖ Place cherry tomatoes in a small bowl, add the olive oil and 1/2 tsp salt, and toss the tomatoes ❖ In the meantime, inspiralize the zucchini, set aside ❖ Pour the pesto over the zucchini noodles, using salad toss or tongs, mix the pesto in with the zoodles until it is completely combined ❖ Place the chicken on the grill and grill each side for 5-7 minutes, or until cooked through ❖ Place cherry tomatoes in a grill basket and grill for 5 minutes, until tomatoes burst ❖ Remove the tomatoes and chicken from the grill, slice the chicken and place both sliced chicken and tomatoes into the pesto zoodles bowl ❖ allow the dish to cool completely ❖ Distribute among the containers, store for 2-3 days ❖ To Serve: Reheat in the microwave for 1-2 minutes or until heated through. Enjoy

222) NIÇOISE-STYLE TUNA SALAD WITH OLIVES AND WHITE BEANS

	Cooking Time: 20-30 Minutes	Servings: 4

Ingredients	Ingredients	Instructions
✓ Green beans (.75 lb.) ✓ Solid white albacore tuna (12 oz. can) ✓ Great Northern beans (16 oz. can) ✓ Sliced black olives (2.25 oz.) ✓ Thinly sliced medium red onion (¼ of 1)	✓ Hard-cooked eggs (4 large) ✓ Dried oregano (1 tsp.) ✓ Olive oil (6 tbsp.) ✓ Black pepper and salt (as desired) ✓ Finely grated lemon zest (.5 tsp.) ✓ Water (.33 cup) ✓ Lemon juice (3 tbsp.)	❖ Drain the can of tuna, Great Northern beans, and black olives. Trim and snap the green beans into halves. Thinly slice the red onion. Cook and peel the eggs until hard-boiled. ❖ Pour the water and salt into a skillet and add the beans. Place a top on the pot and switch the temperature setting to high. Wait for it to boil. ❖ Once the beans are cooking, set a timer for five minutes. Immediately, drain and add the beans to a cookie sheet with a raised edge on paper towels to cool. ❖ Combine the onion, olives, white beans, and drained tuna. Mix them with the zest, lemon juice, oil, and oregano. ❖ Dump the mixture over the salad and gently toss. ❖ Adjust the seasonings to your liking. Portion the tuna-bean salad with the green beans and eggs to serve.

223) WHOLE WHEAT PASTA AND ROASTED RED BELL PEPPER SAUCE WITH FRESH MOZZARELLA CHEES

	Cooking Time: 40 Minutes	Servings: 4

Ingredients	Ingredients	Instructions
✓ 3 large red bell peppers, seeds removed and cut in half ✓ 1 (10-ounce) container cherry tomatoes ✓ 2 tsp olive oil, plus 2 tbsp ✓ 8 ounces whole-wheat penne or rotini	✓ 1 tbsp plus 1 tsp apple cider vinegar ✓ 1 tsp chopped garlic ✓ 1½ tsp smoked paprika ✓ ¼ tsp kosher salt ✓ ½ cup packed fresh basil leaves, chopped ✓ 1 (8-ounce) container fresh whole-milk mozzarella balls (ciliegine), quartered	❖ Preheat the oven to 400°F and line a sheet pan with a silicone baking mat or parchment paper. ❖ Place the peppers and tomatoes on the pan and toss with tsp of oil. Roast for 40 minutes. ❖ While the peppers and tomatoes are roasting, cook the pasta according to the instructions on the box. Drain and place the pasta in a large mixing bowl. ❖ When the peppers are cool enough to handle, peel the skin and discard. It's okay if you can't remove all the skin. Place the roasted peppers, vinegar, garlic, paprika, and salt and the remaining 2 tbsp of oil in a blender and blend until smooth. ❖ Add the pepper sauce, whole roasted tomatoes, basil, and mozzarella to the pasta and stir to combine. ❖ Place a heaping 2 cups of pasta and sauce in each of 4 containers. ❖ STORAGE: Store covered containers in the refrigerator for up to 5 days.

224) GREEK TURKEY MEATBALL GYRO AND TZATZIKI

Cooking Time: 16 Minutes	Servings: 4

- Turkey Meatball:
- 1 lb. ground turkey
- 1/4 cup finely diced red onion
- 2 garlic cloves, minced
- 1 tsp oregano
- 1 cup chopped fresh spinach
- Salt, to taste
- Pepper, to taste
- 2 tbsp olive oil

- Tzatziki Sauce:
- 1/2 cup plain Greek yogurt
- 1/4 cup grated cucumber
- 2 tbsp lemon juice
- 1/2 tsp dry dill
- 1/2 tsp garlic powder
- Salt, to taste
- 1/2 cup thinly sliced red onion
- 1 cup diced tomato
- 1 cup diced cucumber
- 4 whole wheat flatbreads

- In a large bowl, add in ground turkey, diced red onion, oregano, fresh spinach minced garlic, salt, and pepper
- Using your hands mix all the ingredients together until the meat forms a ball and sticks together Then using your hands, form meat mixture into 1" balls, making about 12 meatballs
- In a large skillet over medium high heat, add the olive oil and then add the meatballs, cook each side for 3-minutes until they are browned on all sides, remove from the pan and allow it to rest Allow the dish to cool completely
- Distribute in the container, store for 2-3 days
- To Serve: Reheat in the microwave for 1-2 minutes or until heated through. In the meantime, in a small bowl, combine the Greek yogurt, grated cucumber, lemon juice, dill, garlic powder, and salt to taste Assemble the gyros by taking the toasted flatbread, add 3 meatballs, sliced red onion, tomato, and cucumber. Top with Tzatziki sauce and serve!

Nutrition: Calories:429;Carbs: 3;Total Fat: 19g;Protein: 28g

225) ITALIAN STYLE GRILLED CHICKEN SKEWERS

Cooking Time: 10 Minutes	Servings: 10

- Chicken Kebabs:
- 3 chicken fillets, cut in 1-inch cubes
- 2 red bell peppers
- 2 green bell peppers
- 1 red onion
- Chicken Kebab Marinade:
- 2/3 cup extra virgin olive oil, divided

- Juice of 1 lemon, divided
- 6 clove of garlic, chopped, divided
- 4 tsp salt, divided
- 2 tsp freshly ground black pepper, divided
- 2 tsp paprika, divided
- 2 tsp thyme, divided
- 4 tsp oregano, divided

- In a bowl, mix 2 of all ingredients for the marinade- olive oils, lemon juice, garlic, salt, pepper, paprika, thyme and oregano in small bowl
- Place the chicken in a ziplock bag and pour marinade over it, marinade in the fridge for about 30 minutes
- In a separate ziplock bag, mix the other half of the marinade ingredients - olive oils, lemon juice, garlic, salt, pepper, paprika, thyme and oregano - add the vegetables and marinade for at least minutes
- If you are using wood skewers, soak the skewers in water for about 20-30 minutes
- Once done, thread the chicken and peppers and onions on the skewers in a pattern about 6 pieces of chicken with peppers and onion in between
- Over an outdoor grill or indoor grill pan over medium-high heat, spray the grates lightly with oil
- Grill the chicken for about 5 minutes on each side, or until cooked through, then allow to cool completely. Distribute among the containers, store for 2-3 days. To Serve: Reheat in the microwave for 1-2 minutes or until heated through, or cover in foil and reheat in the oven at 375 degrees F for 5 minutes
- Recipe Notes: You can also bake the Italian-Style chicken skewers in the oven. Just preheat the oven to 425 F and place the chicken skewers on roasting racks that are over two foil-lined baking sheets. Bake for 15 minutes, turn over and bake for an additional 10 - 15 minutes on the other side, or until cooked through

Nutrition: Calories:228;Carbs: 5g;Total Fat: 17g;Protein: 14g

226) CILANTRO KIDNEY BEANS SALAD

	Cooking Time: 30 Minutes	**Servings:** 6

Ingredients:

- ✓ 1 15-ounce can kidney beans, rinsed and drained
- ✓ ½ English cucumber, chopped
- ✓ 1 medium heirloom tomato, chopped
- ✓ 1 bunch fresh cilantro, stems removed and chopped (about 1¼ cups)
- ✓ 1 red onion, chopped
- ✓ lime juice, 1 large lime
- ✓ 3 tbsp Dijon mustard
- ✓ ½ tsp fresh garlic paste
- ✓ 1 tsp sumac
- ✓ salt
- ✓ pepper

Directions:

- ❖ Place kidney beans, vegetables, and cilantro in a serving bowl.
- ❖ Cover, refrigerate and allow it to chill.
- ❖ Before serving, in a small bowl, make the vinaigrette by adding limejuice, oil, fresh garlic, pepper, mustard, and sumac.
- ❖ Pour the vinaigrette over the salad and give it a gentle stir.
- ❖ Add some salt and pepper.
- ❖ Serve!

Nutrition: Calories: 269, Total Fat: 1.3 g, Saturated Fat: 0.2 g, Cholesterol: 0 mg, Sodium: 112 mg, Total Carbohydrate: 49.3 g, Dietary Fiber: 12.g, Total Sugars: 3.9 g, Protein: 17.6 g, Vitamin D: 0 mcg, Calcium: 94 mg, Iron: 6 mg, Potassium: 1258 mg

227) BARLEY WITH MUSHROOM SOUP

	Cooking Time: 30 Minutes	**Servings:** 6

Ingredients:

- ✓ 2 tbsp of olive oil
- ✓ 1 cup chopped carrots
- ✓ 6 cups vegetable broth, no salt added, and low sodium is best
- ✓ ¼ cup red wine
- ✓ 5 tbsp parmesan cheese, grated
- ✓ ½ tsp thyme
- ✓ 1 cup chopped onion
- ✓ 5 cups chopped mushrooms
- ✓ 1 cup pearled barley, uncooked
- ✓ 2 tbsp tomato paste

Directions:

- ❖ Place a stockpot on your stove and turn the temperature of the range to medium heat.
- ❖ Pour in the oil and let it warm up and start to simmer.
- ❖ Combine the carrots and onion. Let them cook for 5 to 8 minutes while frequently stirring the ingredients together.
- ❖ Add the mushroom and turn the heat up to medium-high. Stir and cook for a few minutes.
- ❖ Pour in the broth and stir the ingredients for a few seconds.
- ❖ Add in the wine, barley, thyme, and tomato paste. Stir everything together and then set the cover on the pot.
- ❖ When the soup starts to boil, stir and reduce the heat to medium-low.
- ❖ Cover the soup again and set your timer for 15 minutes, but don't leave it alone. You will want to stir a few times, so all ingredients become well incorporated.
- ❖ Once the dish becomes fragrant and the barley is completely cooked, turn off the heat and serve in bowls. Sprinkle the cheese on top for added taste and enjoy!

Nutrition: calories: 236, fats: 7 grams, carbohydrates: 35 grams, protein: 8 grams.

228) PAN-SEARED SCALLOPS WITH PEPPER AND ONIONS IN ANCHOVY OIL

	Cooking Time: 45 Minutes	Servings: 4

Ingredients:

- ✓ Olive oil (.33 cup)
- ✓ Anchovy fillets (2 oz. can)
- ✓ Jumbo sea scallops (1 lb.)
- ✓ Orange & red bell pepper (1 large of each)
- ✓ Red onion (1)
- ✓ Garlic (2 cloves)
- ✓ Lime zest (1 tsp.)
- ✓ Lemon zest (1.5 tsp.)
- ✓ Kosher salt & pepper (1 pinch of each)
- ✓ Garnish: Fresh parsley (8 sprigs)

Directions:

- ❖ Coarsely chop the peppers and onions. Mince the garlic and anchovy fillet. Zest/mince the lime and lemon.
- ❖ Heat the oil and anchovies in a large skillet using a med-high temperature setting.
- ❖ After the anchovies are sizzling, toss in the scallops, and simmer them for about two minutes - without stirring.
- ❖ Toss the bell peppers, garlic, red onion, lime zest, lemon zest, salt, and pepper into a mixing container. Sprinkle the mixture over the scallops. Cook until they have browned (2 min..)
- ❖ Flip the scallops, stir, and continue cooking until the scallops have browned thoroughly (4-min..)
- ❖ Top it off using sprigs of parsley before serving.

Nutrition: Calories: 368;Protein: 24.2 grams;Fat: 23.9 grams

229) SPECIAL CHICKEN ARTICHOKE, SAUSAGE, KALE, AND WHITE BEAN GRATIN

	Cooking Time: 45 Minutes	Servings: 8

Ingredients:

- ✓ 2 tsp olive oil, plus 2 tbsp
- ✓ 1 small yellow onion, chopped (about 2 cups)
- ✓ 1 (12-ounce) package fully cooked chicken-apple sausage, sliced
- ✓ 1 bunch kale, stemmed and chopped (6 to 7 cups)
- ✓ ½ cup dry white wine, such as sauvignon blanc
- ✓ 4 ounces soft goat cheese
- ✓ 2 (15.5-ounce) cans cannellini or great northern beans, drained and rinsed
- ✓ 1 (14-ounce) can quartered artichoke hearts
- ✓ 1 (14.5-ounce) can no-salt-added diced tomatoes
- ✓ 1 tsp herbes de Provence
- ✓ ¼ tsp kosher salt
- ✓ 1 cup panko bread crumbs
- ✓ 1 tsp garlic powder

Directions:

- ❖ Preheat the oven to 350°F. Lightly oil a -by-9-inch glass or ceramic baking dish.
- ❖ Heat tsp of oil in a 12-inch skillet over medium-high heat. When the oil is shimmering, add the onion and cook for 2 minutes. Add the sausage and brown for 3 minutes. Add the kale and cook until wilted, about 3 more minutes. Add the wine and cook for 1 additional minute.
- ❖ Add the goat cheese and stir until it is melted and the mixture looks creamy. Add the beans, artichokes, tomatoes, herbes de Provence, and salt, and stir to combine. Transfer the contents of the pan to the baking dish.
- ❖ Mix the bread crumbs, the garlic powder, and the remaining 2 tbsp of oil in a small bowl. Spread the bread crumbs evenly across the top of the casserole.
- ❖ Cover the dish with foil and bake for 30 minutes. Remove the foil and bake for 15 more minutes, until the bread crumbs are lightly browned. Cool. Place about 1½ cups of casserole in each of 8 containers.
- ❖ STORAGE: Store covered containers in the refrigerator for up to 5 days. Gratin can be frozen for up to 3 months.

Nutrition: Total calories: 367; Total fat: 14g; Saturated fat: 5g; Sodium: 624mg; Carbohydrates: 40g; Fiber: 10g; Protein: 1

230) EASY ZUCCHINI SALAD WITH POMEGRANATE DRESSING

Preparation Time: 8 minutes	Cooking Time: 15 minutes	Servings: 6

Ingredients:

- ✓ One bunch of chives
- ✓ One pomegranate
- ✓ 1 tbsp pomegranate molasses
- ✓ 1/2 orange juice
- ✓ 1/4 cup mint leaf
- ✓ 120 g feta cheese
- ✓ 2 Lebanese cucumbers
- ✓ 2 tbsp currants
- ✓ 2 tbsp olive oil
- ✓ Three zucchinis
- ✓ salt and pepper

Directions:

- ❖ Clean the zucchini, then cucumber and slice the cucumber and cut it into ribbons using a peeler. And the same thing about your zucchini. Put the cucumber in the fridge.
- ❖ Chop chives into 2cm chunks and chop mint loosely.
- ❖ Make an orange Juice and combine with olive oil, a touch of pepper and salt, and 1 tbsp of pomegranate molasses to make the dressing. Whisk to blend.
- ❖ Toss the cucumber and zucchini into the dressing and apply the sliced herbs to prepare the salad.
- ❖ Add flowers and finish with the crumbled feta cheese.
- ❖ Slice the pomegranate into half and touch the skin's back with the dessert spoon to scatter the seeds over the salad.
- ❖ Now Serve.

Nutrition: Calories: 177.7 kcal Fat: 9.8 g Protein: 5.7 g Carbs: 20 g Fiber: 3.9 g

231) ITALIAN-STYLE GRAIN SALAD

Preparation Time: 5 minutes	Cooking Time: 35 minutes	Servings: 1

Ingredients:

- ✓ Coarse salt to taste
- ✓ Black pepper 2 tsp olive oil 1/2 minced small shallot 1/2 cup parsley, chopped 1
- ✓ 1 tbsp red wine vinegar 1 oz goat cheese, crumbled 1 cup grape tomatoes, halved

Directions:

- ❖ Combine the bulgur with 1/4 tsp salt and 1 cup of boiling water in a heat-proof dish. Cover, and let rest for about 30 minutes, before tender but somewhat chewy.
- ❖ Drain the bulgur and press to extract liquid in the fine-mesh sieve; return to the bowl. Add the onions, parsley, vinegar, shallot, and oil. Then season with pepper and salt, and toss.
- ❖ Top with cheese.

Nutrition: Calories:303 kcal Fat: 21g Protein: 10g Carbs: 21g Fiber: 4g

232) TROPICAL MACADAMIA NUTS DRESSING

Preparation Time: 10 minutes	Cooking Time: 10 minutes	Servings: 4

Ingredients:

- ✓ 1/4 tsp onion powder
- ✓ 1/2 tsp pepper
- ✓ 1 cup Cashew Milk
- ✓ 1 cup Macadamia Nuts
- ✓ 1 tbsp chives, chopped
- ✓ 1 tbsp lemon juice
- ✓ 1 tsp apple cider vinegar
- ✓ 1 tsp garlic powder
- ✓ 1 tsp salt
- ✓ 2 tbsp parsley

Directions:

- ❖ A high-powered mixer and places all the ingredients (other than green onions and chives, and parsley). Start at low and bring it up to high speed steadily until the ingredients are fully blended. If you want a thinner consistency, add more Homemade Cashew Milk from Nature's Eats.
- ❖ Add now the diced chives and parsley, then blend until smooth.
- ❖ Now serve promptly or store it in the refrigerator in an air-tight bag.

Nutrition: Calories: 302 kcal Fat: 26 g Protein: 8 g Carbs: 19 g Fiber: 6.3 g

233) EASY VINAIGRETTE DRESSING

Preparation Time: 5 minutes	Cooking Time: 5 minutes	Servings: 1

✓ black pepper, to taste ✓ 3 tbsp vinegar ✓ Two cloves garlic, minced	✓ 1 tbsp honey ✓ 1 tbsp Dijon mustard ✓ ½ cup olive oil ✓ ¼ tsp salt	❖ Combine all the ingredients in a liquid mixing cup. With a small spoon or a fork, stir well till ingredients are thoroughly mixed together. ❖ Now taste, and customize as needed. Thin it out with a little more olive oil if the mixture becomes too acidic, or balance the flavors with a bit more maple, honey, or syrup. Add a pinch of salt if the mixture is a bit blah. If the zing is not enough, apply a tsp of vinegar. ❖ Serve instantly, or for potential use, cover, and refrigerate. For 7 to 10 days, the homemade vinaigrette lasts well. If the vinaigrette solidifies in the fridge somewhat, don't think about it. It helps to do this with real olive oil. Simply let it for 5 to 10 minutes at room temperature or microwave very quickly (approximately 20 secs) to liquefy that olive oil again. Now serve.

234) Greek style turkey burger with Tzatziki sauce

Preparation Time: 36 minutes	Cooking Time: 10 minutes	Servings: 4

✓ Turkey Burgers ✓ 1 lb ground turkey ✓ 1/3 cup chopped sun-dried tomatoes ✓ ½ cup chopped spinach leaves ✓ 1/4 cup chopped red onion ✓ 2 pressed garlic cloves ✓ ¼ cup feta cheese ✓ One egg ✓ 1 tsp dried oregano ✓ 1 tbsp olive oil ✓ 1/2 tsp kosher salt ✓ One sliced red onion	✓ Four hamburger buns ✓ 1/2 tsp ground black pepper ✓ A handful of Bibb lettuce leaves ✓ Tzatziki Sauce ✓ ½ grated cucumber ✓ Two minced garlic cloves ✓ 3/4 cup Greek yogurt ✓ 1 tbsp red wine vinegar ✓ One pinch of kosher salt ✓ 1 tbsp chopped dill ✓ One pinch of black pepper	❖ Combine all the ingredients of Tzatziki sauce in a bowl and mix well. ❖ Mix turkey, onion, sun-dried tomatoes, and feta cheese in a bowl. ❖ In another bowl, mix olive oil, egg, garlic, salt, oregano, and pepper. ❖ Pour egg mixture with turkey mixture. Mix well. ❖ Make medium-sized patties out of turkey mixture. Set aside in the refrigerator for 24 hours. ❖ Cook turkey patties on heated grill sprayed with oil for seven minutes from both sides on medium flame. ❖ Spread Tzatziki sauce over buns and place lettuce, onions, and cooked patties and serve.

235) SAUCY GREEK-STYLE BAKED SHRIMP

Preparation Time: 15 minutes	Cooking Time: 20 minutes	Servings: 4

✓ 2 tbsp chopped dill ✓ 1 lb shrimp ✓ 1/4 tsp kosher salt ✓ 1/2 tsp red pepper flakes ✓ 3 tbsp olive oil ✓ Three minced garlic cloves	✓ One chopped onion ✓ 15 oz crushed tomatoes ✓ 1/2 tsp ground cinnamon ✓ 1/2 tsp ground allspice ✓ 1/2 cup crumbled feta cheese	❖ Add salt, shrimps, and pepper in a bowl. Toss well and keep it aside. ❖ Cook garlic and onions in heated olive oil over medium flame for five minutes. ❖ Add spices and stir for half a minute. ❖ Mix tomatoes and let it simmer for 20 minutes with occasional stirring. ❖ Transfer the tomato mixture to the baking sheet and add shrimps to it. Spread cheese and bake in a preheated oven at 375 degrees for 20 minutes. ❖ Drizzle dill and serve.

Nutrition: Calories: 190 kcal Fat: 5.2 g Protein: 25.9 g Carbs: 11.9 g Fiber: 5.2 g

236) TASTY SAUTÉED CHICKEN WITH OLIVES CAPERS AND LEMONS

Preparation Time: 5 minutes	Cooking Time: 30 minutes	Servings: 4

Ingredients:

- ✓ Six boneless chicken thighs
- ✓ Two sliced lemons
- ✓ One minced garlic clove minced
- ✓ 2/4 cup extra virgin olive oil
- ✓ 2 tbsp all-purpose flour
- ✓ 2 tbsp butter
- ✓ 1 cup chicken broth
- ✓ kosher salt to taste
- ✓ 3/4 cup Sicilian green olives
- ✓ 2 tbsp parsley
- ✓ 1/4 cup capers
- ✓ Black pepper to taste

Directions:

- ❖ Add salt, chicken, and pepper in a bowl and toss well. Set aside for 15 minutes.
- ❖ Cook lemon slices (half of them) in heated olive oil over medium flame for five minutes from both sides.
- ❖ Shift the cooked brown lemon slices on the plate.
- ❖ Coat chicken pieces with rice flour and cook in heated olive oil in the skillet for seven minutes from both sides. Transfer the cooked chicken to the plate.
- ❖ Sauté garlic in heated oil in the same pan for about half a minute. Stir in olives, chicken broth, lemons, and capers. Cook over high flame for few minutes.
- ❖ When half of the broth is left, add parsley and butter. Cook for one minute.
- ❖ Add salt and pepper to adjust the taste and serve.

Nutrition: Calories: 595 kcal Fat: 34 g Protein: 51 g Carbs: 5.5 g Fiber: 9 g

237) ENGLISH PORRIDGE (OATMEAL)

Preparation Time: 2 minutes	Cooking Time: 2 minutes	Servings: 1

Ingredients:

- ✓ Base Recipe
- ✓ ½ cup oats
- ✓ 1/2cup water
- ✓ 1/2cup milk
- ✓ 1 Pinch salt
- ✓ Maple Brown Sugar
- ✓ 1 tsp sugar
- ✓ 2 tbsp chopped pecans
- ✓ 1 tsp maple syrup
- ✓ 1/8 tsp cinnamon
- ✓ Banana Nut
- ✓ ½ banana sliced
- ✓ 1 tbsp flaxseed
- ✓ 2 tbsp walnuts
- ✓ 1/8 tsp cinnamon
- ✓ Strawberry & Cream
- ✓ 1/2cup strawberries
- ✓ 2 tsp honey
- ✓ 1 tbsp half and half
- ✓ 1/8 tsp vanilla extract
- ✓ Chocolate Peanut Butter
- ✓ 2 tsp cocoa powder
- ✓ 2 tsp chocolate chips
- ✓ 1 tbsp peanut butter
- ✓ 1 tsp roasted peanuts

Directions:

- ❖ Microwave Instructions
- ❖ Place all the ingredients heat in the microwave on high for 2 minutes. Then add 15-sec increments until the oatmeal is puffed and softened.
- ❖ Stovetop Instructions
- ❖ Bring the water and milk to a boil in a pan. Lower the heat & pour in the oats. Cook it while stirring, till the oats are soft and have absorbed most of the liquid.Turn off the stove and let it for 2 to 3 min.
- ❖ Assembly
- ❖ Stir in the toppings and let rest for a few minutes to cool. Serve warm.

Nutrition: Calories: 227 kcal Fat:6 g Protein: 9 g Carbs: 33 g Fiber: 4 g

238) MOROCCAN SALAD FATTOUSH

Preparation Time: 20 minutes	Cooking Time: 20 minutes	Servings: 6

Ingredients:

- ✓ Two loaves of pita bread
- ✓ • ½ tsp sumac
- ✓ • Olive Oil
- ✓ • Salt and pepper
- ✓ • One chopped English cucumber
- ✓ • One chopped lettuce
- ✓ • Five chopped Roma tomatoes
- ✓ Five radishes
- ✓ • Five chopped green onions
- ✓ • 2 cup parsley leaves
- ✓ Lime-vinaigrette
- ✓ • 1/4 tsp cinnamon
- ✓ • 1 tsp lime juice
- ✓ • Salt and pepper
- ✓ • 1/3 cup Virgin Olive Oil
- ✓ • 1 tsp sumac
- ✓ • 1/4 tsp allspice

Directions:

- ❖ Toast the bread in the oven. Heat olive oil and fry until browned. Add salt, pepper, and 1/2tsp of sumac. Turn off heat & place pita chips on paper towels to drain.
- ❖ In a mixing bowl, mix the chopped lettuce, cucumber, tomatoes, green onions with the sliced radish and parsley.
- ❖ For seasoning, whisk the lemon or lime juice, olive oil, and spices in a small bowl.
- ❖ Sprinkle the salad & toss lightly. Finally, add the pita chips and more sumac if you like. Shifts to small serving bowls or plates. Enjoy!

Nutrition: Calories: 345 kcal Fat:20.4 g Protein: 9.1 g Carbs:39.8 g Fiber: 1 g

239) CALABRIA CICORIA E FAGIOLI

Preparation Time:	Cooking Time:	Servings: 6

Ingredients:

- ✓ 200 g dried cannellini beans
- ✓ • 6 tbsp olive oil
- ✓ • 400 g curly endive
- ✓ Four garlic cloves
- ✓ • 600 ml of water
- ✓ • Two red chilies
- ✓ • Salt and pepper to taste

Directions:

- ❖ Put the dried beans to soak for 12 h (they increase in size). Drain them and boil for two h in fresh unsalted water. Salt at the end of the cooking time. If using canned beans, drain them from their liquid and rinse them before use. Rinse the endive and cut it up into short lengths.
- ❖ Heat the olive oil, fry the garlic without browning, and then add the endive and chilies. Keeping the heat high, stir-fry for a minute or two, coating the endive with the oil, then add the drained cannellini beans, some salt, and the water. Bring to the boil, cover the pan, and lower the heat. Cook until the endive is soft and most of the liquid has been absorbed.

Nutrition: Calories:225 kcal Fat: 21 g Protein: 3 g Carbs: 6 g Fiber:1 g

240) CAMPANIA POACHED EGGS CAPRESE

Preparation Time: 10 minutes	Cooking Time: 10 minutes	Servings: 2

Ingredients:

- ✓ 4 tsp pesto
- ✓ • 1 tbsp white vinegar
- ✓ • Four eggs
- ✓ • 2 tsp salt
- ✓ 2 English muffins
- ✓ • salt to taste
- ✓ • One tomato sliced
- ✓ • Four slices of mozzarella cheese

Directions:

❖ Fill 2 to 3 inches of a pan with water and boil over a high flame. Lower the heat, add the vinegar, 2 tsp of salt in it, and let it simmer.

❖ Put a cheese slice and a slice of tomato on every English muffin half and put in a toaster oven for 5 min or till the cheese melts and the English muffin is well toasted.

❖ Break an egg in a bowl and add in the water one by one. Let the eggs cook for 2.5 to 3 minutes or until the yolks have solidified and the egg whites are firm. Take the eggs out of the water and put them on a kitchen towel to absorb excess water.

❖ For assembling, first put an egg on top of every muffin, add a tsp of pesto sauce on the egg, and scatter the salt.

241) GREEK BREAKFAST DISH WITH EGGS AND VEGETABLES

Preparation Time: 10 minutes	Cooking Time: 10 minutes	Servings: 2

Ingredients:

- ✓ 1 tbsp olive oil
- ✓ • salt to taste
- ✓ • 2 cup chopped rainbow chard
- ✓ • ½ cup arugula
- ✓ 1 cup spinach
- ✓ • Two cloves garlic
- ✓ • ½ cup grated Cheddar cheese
- ✓ • Four eggs
- ✓ • black pepper to taste

Directions:

❖ Heat oil over moderate pressure. Sauté the chard, spinach, and arugula until soft, around three minutes. Add garlic, continue cooking until aromatic, approx. Two min.

❖ In a cup, combine the eggs and the cheese; dump into the mixture of the chard. Heat and cook for 5 - 6 minutes. Season to taste with salt and pepper.

242) ITALIAN BREAKFAST PITA PIZZA

Preparation Time: 25 minutes	Cooking Time: 30 minutes	Servings: 2

Ingredients:

- ✓ Four slices of bacon
- ✓ 2 tbsp olive oil
- ✓ 1/4 onion
- ✓ Four eggs
- ✓ Two pita bread rounds
- ✓ 2 tbsp pesto
- ✓ ½ tomato
- ✓ One avocado
- ✓ ½ cup slashed spinach
- ✓ 1/4 cup mushrooms
- ✓ ½ cup grated Cheddar cheese

Directions:

❖ Heat the oven to 350 ° F (175° C).

❖ In a medium saucepan, put the bacon and cook over medium-high heat, rotating periodically, when browned uniformly, around ten minutes. Cook the onion in the same skillet till smooth. Put it aside. In the skillet, melt the olive oil. Add the eggs and cook, stirring regularly, for 3 to 5 minutes.

❖ Add the pita bread to the cake pan. Cover with bacon, fried eggs, onions, mushrooms, and spinach; sprinkle the pesto over through the pita. Dress over the toppings of Cheddar cheese.

❖ Bake it in the preheated oven for10 min. Serve with avocado pieces.

243) NAPOLI CAPRESE ON TOAST

Preparation Time: 15 minutes	Cooking Time: 5 minutes	Servings: 14

Ingredients:

- ✓ 14 slices bread
- ✓ 1 lb mozzarella cheese
- ✓ Two cloves garlic
- ✓ 1/3 cup basil leaves
- ✓ 3 tbsp olive oil
- ✓ Three tomatoes
- ✓ salt to taste
- ✓ black pepper to taste

Directions:

❖ Baked the bread slices and spread the garlic on one side of each piece. Put a slice of mozzarella cheese, 1 to 2 basil leaves, and a slice of tomato on each piece of toast. Sprinkle with olive oil, spray salt, and black pepper.

Nutrition: Calories: 203.5 kcal Fat: 10 g Protein: 10.5 g Carbs: 16.5 g Fiber: 1.1 g

244) TUSCAN EGGS FLORENTINE

Preparation Time: 10 minutes	Cooking Time: 10 minutes	Servings: 3

Ingredients:

- ✓ 2 tbsp butter
- ✓ Two cloves garlic
- ✓ 3 tbsp cream cheese
- ✓ ½ cup mushroom
- ✓ ½ fresh spinach
- ✓ Salt to taste
- ✓ Six eggs
- ✓ Black pepper to taste

Directions:

- ❖ Put the butter in a non-stick skillet; heat and mix the mushrooms and garlic till the garlic is flavorsome for about 1 min. Add spinach to the mushroom paste and cook until spinach is softened for 2 - 3 mins,
- ❖ Mix the mushroom-spinach mixer; add salt and pepper. Cook, with mixing, until the eggs are stiff; turn. Pour with cream cheese over the egg mixture and cook before cream cheese started melting just over five minutes.

Nutrition: Calories: 278.9 kcal Fat: 22.9 g Protein:15.7 g Carbs: 4.1 g Fiber:22.9

245) SPECIAL QUINOA, CEREALS FOR BREAKFAST

Preparation Time: 5 minutes	Cooking Time: 16 minutes	Servings: 4

Ingredients:

- ✓ 2 cups of water
- ✓ ½ cup apricots
- ✓ 1 cup quinoa
- ✓ ½ cup almonds
- ✓ 1 tsp cinnamon
- ✓ 1/3 cup seeds
- ✓ ½ tsp nutmeg

Directions:

- ❖ Combine water and quinoa in a medium saucepan and continue cooking. Lower the heat and boil when much of the water has been drained for 8–12 minutes. Whisk in apricots, almonds, linseeds, cinnamon, and nutmeg; simmer till the quinoa is soft.

Nutrition: Calories: 349.9 kcal Fat:15.1 g Protein: 11.8 g Carbs: 44.5 g Fiber: 9.3 g

246) SIMPLE ZUCCHINI WITH EGG

Preparation Time: 5 minutes	Cooking Time: 15 minutes	Servings: 2

Ingredients:

- ✓ Two eggs
- ✓ 1.5 tbsp olive oil
- ✓ salt to taste
- ✓ Two zucchinis
- ✓ Black pepper to taste
- ✓ 1 tsp water

Directions:

- ❖ Heat the oil in a saucepan over medium heat; sauté the zucchini until soft, around 10 minutes. Season with salt and black pepper.
- ❖ Add the eggs with a fork in a bowl; add more water and mix until uniformly mixed. Spill the eggs over the zucchini; continue cooking until the eggs are boiled and rubbery for almost 5 minutes. Dress it with salt and black pepper.

Nutrition: Calories: 21.7 kcal Fat: 15.7 g Protein: 10.2 g Carbs: 11.2 g Fiber: 3.6 g

247) ITALIAN BAKED EGGS IN AVOCADO

Preparation Time: 10 minutes	Cooking Time: 15 minutes	Servings: 2

- ✓ One pinch parsley
- ✓ Two eggs
- ✓ Two slice bacon
- ✓ One avocado
- ✓ 2 tsp chives
- ✓ One pinch of salt and black pepper

Directions:

- ❖ Preheat the oven to 425 degrees.
- ❖ Break the eggs in a tub, willing to maintain the yolks preserved.
- ❖ Assemble the avocado halves in the baking bowl, rest them on the side. Slowly spoon one egg yolk in the avocado opening. Keep spooning the white egg into the hole till it is finished. Do the same with leftover egg yolk, egg white, and avocado. Dress with chives, parsley, sea salt, and pepper for each of the avocados.
- ❖ Gently put the baking dish in the preheated oven and cook for about 15 min well before the eggs are cooked. Sprinkle with bacon over the avocado.

248)　SPECIAL GROUND PORK SKILLET

	Cooking Time: 25 Minutes	Servings: 4

✓ 1 ½ pounds ground pork ✓ 2 tbsp olive oil ✓ 1 bunch kale, trimmed and roughly chopped ✓ 1 cup onions, sliced ✓ 1/4 tsp black pepper, or more to taste	✓ 1/4 cup tomato puree ✓ 1 bell pepper, chopped ✓ 1 tsp sea salt ✓ 1 cup chicken bone broth ✓ 1/4 cup port wine ✓ 2 cloves garlic, pressed ✓ 1 chili pepper, sliced	❖ Heat tbsp of the olive oil in a cast-iron skillet over a moderately high heat. Now, sauté the onion, garlic, and peppers until they are tender and fragrant; reserve. ❖ Heat the remaining tbsp of olive oil; once hot, cook the ground pork and approximately 5 minutes until no longer pink. ❖ Add in the other ingredients and continue to cook for 15 to 17 minutes or until cooked through. ❖ Storing ❖ Place the ground pork mixture in airtight containers or Ziploc bags; keep in your refrigerator for up to 3 to 4 days. ❖ For freezing, place the ground pork mixture in airtight containers or heavy-duty freezer bags. Freeze up to 2 to 3 months. Defrost in the refrigerator. Bon appétit!

Nutrition: 349 Calories, 13g Fat; 4 4g Carbs; 45.3g Protein; 1.2g Fiber

249)　DELICIOUS GREEK STYLE CHEESE PORK

	Cooking Time: 20 Minutes	Servings: 6

✓ 1 tbsp sesame oil ✓ 1 ½ pounds pork shoulder, cut into strips ✓ Himalayan salt and freshly ground black pepper, to taste ✓ 1/2 tsp cayenne pepper ✓ 1/2 cup shallots, roughly chopped	✓ 2 bell peppers, sliced ✓ 1/4 cup cream of onion soup ✓ 1/2 tsp Sriracha sauce ✓ 1 tbsp tahini (sesame butter ✓ 1 tbsp soy sauce ✓ 4 ounces gouda cheese, cut into small pieces	❖ Heat he sesame oil in a wok over a moderately high flame. ❖ Stir-fry the pork strips for 3 to 4 minutes or until just browned on all sides. Add in the spices, shallots and bell peppers and continue to cook for a further 4 minutes. ❖ Stir in the cream of onion soup, Sriracha, sesame butter, and soy sauce; continue to cook for to 4 minutes more. ❖ Top with the cheese and continue to cook until the cheese has melted. ❖ Storing ❖ Place your stir-fry in six airtight containers or Ziploc bags; keep in your refrigerator for 3 to 4 days. ❖ For freezing, wrap tightly with heavy-duty aluminum foil or freezer wrap. It will maintain the best quality for 2 to 3 months. Defrost in the refrigerator and reheat in your wok.

Nutrition: 424 Calories; 29.4g Fat; 3. Carbs; 34.2g Protein; 0.6g Fiber

250)　SPECIAL PORK IN BLUE CHEESE SAUCE

	Cooking Time: 30 Minutes	Servings: 6

✓ 2 pounds pork center cut loin roast, boneless and cut into 6 pieces ✓ 1 tbsp coconut aminos ✓ 6 ounces blue cheese ✓ 1/3 cup heavy cream ✓ 1/3 cup port wine	✓ 1/3 cup roasted vegetable broth, preferably homemade ✓ 1 tsp dried hot chile flakes ✓ 1 tsp dried rosemary ✓ 1 tbsp lard ✓ 1 shallot, chopped ✓ 2 garlic cloves, chopped ✓ Salt and freshly cracked black peppercorns, to taste	❖ Rub each piece of the pork with salt, black peppercorns, and rosemary. ❖ Melt the lard in a saucepan over a moderately high flame. Sear the pork on all sides about 15 minutes; set aside. ❖ Cook the shallot and garlic until they've softened. Add in port wine to scrape up any brown bits from the bottom. ❖ Reduce the heat to medium-low and add in the remaining ingredients; continue to simmer until the sauce has thickened and reduced. ❖ Storing ❖ Divide the pork and sauce into six portions; place each portion in a separate airtight container or Ziploc bag; keep in your refrigerator for 3 to 4 days. ❖ Freeze the pork and sauce in airtight containers or heavy-duty freezer bags. Freeze up to 4 months. Defrost in the refrigerator. Bon appétit!

Nutrition: 34Calories; 18.9g Fat; 1.9g Carbs; 40.3g Protein; 0.3g Fiber

251) MISSISSIPPI-STYLE PULLED PORK

Cooking Time: 6 Hours		Servings: 4

Ingredients	Ingredients	Directions
✓ 1 ½ pounds pork shoulder ✓ 1 tbsp liquid smoke sauce ✓ 1 tsp chipotle powder	✓ Au Jus gravy seasoning packet ✓ 2 onions, cut into wedges ✓ Kosher salt and freshly ground black pepper, taste	❖ Mix the liquid smoke sauce, chipotle powder, Au Jus gravy seasoning packet, salt and pepper. Rub the spice mixture into the pork on all sides. ❖ Wrap in plastic wrap and let it marinate in your refrigerator for 3 hours. ❖ Prepare your grill for indirect heat. Place the pork butt roast on the grate over a drip pan and top with onions; cover the grill and cook for about 6 hours. ❖ Transfer the pork to a cutting board. Now, shred the meat into bite-sized pieces using two forks. ❖ Storing ❖ Divide the pork between four airtight containers or Ziploc bags; keep in your refrigerator for up to 3 to 5 days. ❖ For freezing, place the pork in airtight containers or heavy-duty freezer bags. Freeze up to 4 months. Defrost in the refrigerator. Bon appétit!

252) SPICY WITH CHEESY TURKEY DIP

Cooking Time: 25 Minutes		Servings: 4

Ingredients	Ingredients	Directions
✓ 1 Fresno chili pepper, deveined and minced ✓ 1 ½ cups Ricotta cheese, creamed, 4% fat, softened ✓ 1/4 cup sour cream ✓ 1 tbsp butter, room temperature ✓ 1 shallot, chopped	✓ 1 tsp garlic, pressed ✓ 1 pound ground turkey ✓ 1/2 cup goat cheese, shredded ✓ Salt and black pepper, to taste ✓ 1 ½ cups Gruyère, shredded	❖ Melt the butter in a frying pan over a moderately high flame. Now, sauté the onion and garlic until they have softened. ❖ Stir in the ground turkey and continue to cook until it is no longer pink. ❖ Transfer the sautéed mixture to a lightly greased baking dish. Add in Ricotta, sour cream, goat cheese, salt, pepper, and chili pepper. ❖ Top with the shredded Gruyère cheese. Bake in the preheated oven at 350 degrees F for about 20 minutes or until hot and bubbly in top. ❖ Storing ❖ Place your dip in an airtight container; keep in your refrigerator for up 3 to 4 days. Enjoy!

Nutrition: 284 Calories; 19g Fat; 3.2g Carbs; 26. Protein; 1.6g Fiber

253) TURKEY CHORIZO AND BOK CHOY

Cooking Time: 50 Minutes		Servings: 4

Ingredients	Ingredients	Directions
✓ 4 mild turkey Chorizo, sliced ✓ 1/2 cup full-fat milk ✓ 6 ounces Gruyère cheese, preferably freshly grated ✓ 1 yellow onion, chopped	✓ Coarse salt and ground black pepper, to taste ✓ 1 pound Bok choy, tough stem ends trimmed ✓ 1 cup cream of mushroom soup ✓ 1 tbsp lard, room temperature	❖ Melt the lard in a nonstick skillet over a moderate flame; cook the Chorizo sausage for about 5 minutes, stirring occasionally to ensure even cooking; reserve. ❖ Add in the onion, salt, pepper, Bok choy, and cream of mushroom soup. Continue to cook for 4 minutes longer or until the vegetables have softened. ❖ Spoon the mixture into a lightly oiled casserole dish. Top with the reserved Chorizo. ❖ In a mixing bowl, thoroughly combine the milk and cheese. Pour the cheese mixture over the sausage. ❖ Cover with foil and bake at 36degrees F for about 35 minutes. ❖ Storing ❖ Cut your casserole into four portions. Place each portion in an airtight container; keep in your refrigerator for 3 to 4 days. ❖ For freezing, wrap your portions tightly with heavy-duty aluminum foil or freezer wrap. Freeze up to 1 to 2 months. Defrost in the refrigerator. Enjoy!

254) CLASSIC SPICY CHICKEN BREASTS

Cooking Time: 30 Minutes		Servings: 6

✓ 1 ½ pounds chicken breasts ✓ 1 bell pepper, deveined and chopped ✓ 1 leek, chopped ✓ 1 tomato, pureed ✓ 2 tbsp coriander	✓ 2 garlic cloves, minced ✓ 1 tsp cayenne pepper ✓ 1 tsp dry thyme ✓ 1/4 cup coconut aminos ✓ Sea salt and ground black pepper, to taste	❖ Rub each chicken breasts with the garlic, cayenne pepper, thyme, salt and black pepper. Cook the chicken in a saucepan over medium-high heat. ❖ Sear for about 5 minutes until golden brown on all sides. ❖ Fold in the tomato puree and coconut aminos and bring it to a boil. Add in the pepper, leek, and coriander. ❖ Reduce the heat to simmer. Continue to cook, partially covered, for about 20 minutes. ❖ Storing ❖ Place the chicken breasts in airtight containers or Ziploc bags; keep in your refrigerator for 3 to 4 days. ❖ For freezing, place the chicken breasts in airtight containers or heavy-duty freezer bags. It will maintain the best quality for about 4 months. Defrost in the refrigerator. Bon appétit!

255) DELICIOUS SAUCY BOSTON BUTT

Cooking Time: 1 Hour 20 Minutes		Servings: 8

✓ 1 tbsp lard, room temperature ✓ 2 pounds Boston butt, cubed ✓ Salt and freshly ground pepper ✓ 1/2 tsp mustard powder ✓ A bunch of spring onions, chopped	✓ 2 garlic cloves, minced ✓ 1/2 tbsp ground cardamom ✓ 2 tomatoes, pureed ✓ 1 bell pepper, deveined and chopped ✓ 1 jalapeno pepper, deveined and finely chopped ✓ 1/2 cup unsweetened coconut milk ✓ 2 cups chicken bone broth	❖ In a wok, melt the lard over moderate heat. Season the pork belly with salt, pepper and mustard powder. ❖ Sear the pork for 8 to 10 minutes, stirring periodically to ensure even cooking; set aside, keeping it warm. ❖ In the same wok, sauté the spring onions, garlic, and cardamom. Spoon the sautéed vegetables along with the reserved pork into the slow cooker. ❖ Add in the remaining ingredients, cover with the lid and cook for 1 hour 10 minutes over low heat. ❖ Divide the pork and vegetables between airtight containers or Ziploc bags; keep in your refrigerator for up to 3 to 5 days. ❖ For freezing, place the pork and vegetables in airtight containers or heavy-duty freezer bags. Freeze up to 4 months. Defrost in the refrigerator. Bon appétit!

256) SPECIAL OLD-FASHIONED HUNGARIAN GOULASH

Cooking Time: 9 Hours 10 Minutes		Servings: 4

✓ 1 ½ pounds pork butt, chopped ✓ 1 tsp sweet Hungarian paprika ✓ 2 Hungarian hot peppers, deveined and minced ✓ 1 cup leeks, chopped ✓ 1 ½ tbsp lard ✓ 1 tsp caraway seeds, ground ✓ 4 cups vegetable broth ✓ 2 garlic cloves, crushed ✓ 1 tsp cayenne pepper ✓ 2 cups tomato sauce with herbs	✓ 1 ½ pounds pork butt, chopped ✓ 1 tsp sweet Hungarian paprika ✓ 2 Hungarian hot peppers, deveined and minced ✓ 1 cup leeks, chopped ✓ 1 ½ tbsp lard ✓ 1 tsp caraway seeds, ground ✓ 4 cups vegetable broth ✓ 2 garlic cloves, crushed ✓ 1 tsp cayenne pepper ✓ 2 cups tomato sauce with herbs	❖ Melt the lard in a heavy-bottomed pot over medium-high heat. Sear the pork for 5 to 6 minutes until just browned on all sides; set aside. ❖ Add in the leeks and garlic; continue to cook until they have softened. ❖ Place the reserved pork along with the sautéed mixture in your crock pot. Add in the other ingredients and stir to combine. ❖ Cover with the lid and slow cook for 9 hours on the lowest setting. ❖ Storing ❖ Spoon your goulash into four airtight containers or Ziploc bags; keep in your refrigerator for up to 3 to 4 days. ❖ For freezing, place the goulash in airtight containers. Freeze up to 4 to 6 months. Defrost in the refrigerator. Enjoy!

257) TYPICAL ITALIAN-STYLE CHEESY PORK LOIN

Cooking Time: 25 Minutes	Servings: 4

Ingredients:

- ✓ 1 pound pork loin, cut into 1-inch-thick pieces
- ✓ 1 tsp Italian seasoning mix
- ✓ Salt and pepper, to taste
- ✓ 1 onion, sliced
- ✓ 1 tsp fresh garlic, smashed
- ✓ 2 tbsp black olives, pitted and sliced
- ✓ 2 tbsp balsamic vinegar
- ✓ 1/2 cup Romano cheese, grated
- ✓ 2 tbsp butter, room temperature
- ✓ 1 tbsp curry paste
- ✓ 1 cup roasted vegetable broth
- ✓ 1 tbsp oyster sauce

Directions:

- ❖ In a frying pan, melt the butter over a moderately high heat. Once hot, cook the pork until browned on all sides; season with salt and black pepper and set aside.
- ❖ In the pan drippings, cook the onion and garlic for 4 to 5 minutes or until they've softened.
- ❖ Add in the Italian seasoning mix, curry paste, and vegetable broth. Continue to cook until the sauce has thickened and reduced slightly or about 10 minutes. Add in the remaining ingredients along with the reserved pork.
- ❖ Top with cheese and cook for 10 minutes longer or until cooked through.
- ❖ Storing
- ❖ Divide the pork loin between four airtight containers; keep in your refrigerator for 3 to 5 days.
- ❖ For freezing, place the pork loin in airtight containers or heavy-duty freezer bags. Freeze up to 4 to 6 months. Defrost in the refrigerator. Enjoy!

258) BAKED SPARE RIBS

Cooking Time: 3 Hour 40 Minutes	Servings: 6

Ingredients:

- ✓ 2 pounds spare ribs
- ✓ 1 garlic clove, minced
- ✓ 1 tsp dried marjoram
- ✓ 1 lime, halved
- ✓ Salt and ground black pepper, to taste

Directions:

- ❖ Toss all ingredients in a ceramic dish.
- ❖ Cover and let it refrigerate for 5 to 6 hours.
- ❖ Roast the foil-wrapped ribs in the preheated oven at 275 degrees F degrees for about hours 30 minutes.
- ❖ Storing
- ❖ Divide the ribs into six portions. Place each portion of ribs in an airtight container; keep in your refrigerator for 3 to days.
- ❖ For freezing, place the ribs in airtight containers or heavy-duty freezer bags. Freeze up to 4 to months. Defrost in the refrigerator and reheat in the preheated oven. Bon appétit!

259) HEALTHY CHICKEN PARMESAN SALAD

Cooking Time: 20 Minutes	Servings: 6

- ✓ 2 romaine hearts, leaves separated
- ✓ Flaky sea salt and ground black pepper, to taste
- ✓ 1/4 tsp chili pepper flakes
- ✓ 1 tsp dried basil
- ✓ 1/4 cup Parmesan, finely grated
- ✓ 2 chicken breasts
- ✓ 2 Lebanese cucumbers, sliced
- ✓ For the dressing:
- ✓ 2 large egg yolks
- ✓ 1 tsp Dijon mustard
- ✓ 1 tbsp fresh lemon juice
- ✓ 1/4 cup olive oil
- ✓ 2 garlic cloves, minced

Directions:

- ❖ In a grilling pan, cook the chicken breast until no longer pink or until a meat thermometer registers 5 degrees F. Slice the chicken into strips.
- ❖ Storing
- ❖ Place the chicken breasts in airtight containers or Ziploc bags; keep in your refrigerator for to 4 days.
- ❖ For freezing, place the chicken breasts in airtight containers or heavy-duty freezer bags. It will maintain the best quality for about months. Defrost in the refrigerator.
- ❖ Toss the chicken with the other ingredients. Prepare the dressing by whisking all the ingredients.
- ❖ Dress the salad and enjoy! Keep the salad in your refrigerator for 3 to 5 days.

260) CLASSIC TURKEY WINGS WITH GRAVY SAUCE

Cooking Time: 6 Hours	Servings: 6

Ingredients:

- ✓ 2 pounds turkey wings
- ✓ 1/2 tsp cayenne pepper
- ✓ 4 garlic cloves, sliced
- ✓ 1 large onion, chopped
- ✓ Salt and pepper, to taste
- ✓ 1 tsp dried marjoram
- ✓ 1 tbsp butter, room temperature
- ✓ 1 tbsp Dijon mustard
- ✓ For the Gravy:
- ✓ 1 cup double cream
- ✓ Salt and black pepper, to taste
- ✓ 1/2 stick butter
- ✓ 3/4 tsp guar gum

Directions:

- ❖ Rub the turkey wings with the Dijon mustard and tbsp of butter. Preheat a grill pan over medium-high heat.
- ❖ Sear the turkey wings for 10 minutes on all sides.
- ❖ Transfer the turkey to your Crock pot; add in the garlic, onion, salt, pepper, marjoram, and cayenne pepper. Cover and cook on low setting for 6 hours.
- ❖ Melt 1/2 stick of the butter in a frying pan. Add in the cream and whisk until cooked through.
- ❖ Next, stir in the guar gum, salt, and black pepper along with cooking juices. Let it cook until the sauce has reduced by half.
- ❖ Storing
- ❖ Wrap the turkey wings in foil before packing them into airtight containers; keep in your refrigerator for up to 3 to 4 days.
- ❖ For freezing, place the turkey wings in airtight containers or heavy-duty freezer bags. Freeze up to 2 to 3 months. Defrost in the refrigerator.
- ❖ Keep your gravy in refrigerator for up to 2 days.

261) AUTHENTIC PORK CHOPS WITH HERBS

Cooking Time: 20 Minutes	Servings: 4

Ingredients:

- ✓ 1 tbsp butter
- ✓ 1 pound pork chops
- ✓ 2 rosemary sprigs, minced
- ✓ 1 tsp dried marjoram
- ✓ 1 tsp dried parsley
- ✓ A bunch of spring onions, roughly chopped
- ✓ 1 thyme sprig, minced
- ✓ 1/2 tsp granulated garlic
- ✓ 1/2 tsp paprika, crushed
- ✓ Coarse salt and ground black pepper, to taste

- ❖ Season the pork chops with the granulated garlic, paprika, salt, and black pepper.
- ❖ Melt the butter in a frying pan over a moderate flame. Cook the pork chops for 6 to 8 minutes, turning them occasionally to ensure even cooking.
- ❖ Add in the remaining ingredients and cook an additional 4 minutes.
- ❖ Storing
- ❖ Divide the pork chops into four portions; place each portion in a separate airtight container or Ziploc bag; keep in your refrigerator for 3 to 4 days.
- ❖ Freeze the pork chops in airtight containers or heavy-duty freezer bags. Freeze up to 4 months. Defrost in the refrigerator. Bon appétit!

262) PEPPERS STUFFED WITH CHOPPED PORK ORIGINAL

Cooking Time: 40 Minutes	Servings: 4

Ingredients:

- ✓ 6 bell peppers, deveined
- ✓ 1 tbsp vegetable oil
- ✓ 1 shallot, chopped
- ✓ 1 garlic clove, minced
- ✓ 1/2 pound ground pork
- ✓ 1/3 pound ground veal
- ✓ 1 ripe tomato, chopped
- ✓ 1/2 tsp mustard seeds
- ✓ Sea salt and ground black pepper, to taste

- ❖ Parboil the peppers for 5 minutes.
- ❖ Heat the vegetable oil in a frying pan that is preheated over a moderate heat. Cook the shallot and garlic for 3 to 4 minutes until they've softened.
- ❖ Stir in the ground meat and cook, breaking apart with a fork, for about 6 minutes. Add the chopped tomatoes, mustard seeds, salt, and pepper.
- ❖ Continue to cook for 5 minutes or until heated through. Divide the filling between the peppers and transfer them to a baking pan.
- ❖ Bake in the preheated oven at 36degrees F approximately 25 minutes.
- ❖ Storing
- ❖ Place the peppers in airtight containers or Ziploc bags; keep in your refrigerator for up to 3 to 4 days.
- ❖ For freezing, place the peppers in airtight containers or heavy-duty freezer bags. Freeze up to 2 to 3 months. Defrost in the refrigerator. Bon appétit!

Nutrition: 2 Calories; 20.5g Fat; 8.2g Carbs; 18.2g Protein; 1.5g Fiber

263) GRILL-STYLE CHICKEN SALAD WITH AVOCADO

	Cooking Time: 20 Minutes	Servings: 4

Ingredients:

- ✓ 1/3 cup olive oil
- ✓ 2 chicken breasts
- ✓ Sea salt and crushed red pepper flakes
- ✓ 2 egg yolks
- ✓ 1 tbsp fresh lemon juice
- ✓ 1/2 tsp celery seeds
- ✓ 1 tbsp coconut aminos
- ✓ 1 large-sized avocado, pitted and sliced

Directions:

- ❖ Grill the chicken breasts for about 4 minutes per side. Season with salt and pepper, to taste.
- ❖ Slice the grilled chicken into bite-sized strips.
- ❖ To make the dressing, whisk the egg yolks, lemon juice, celery seeds, olive oil and coconut aminos in a measuring cup.
- ❖ Storing
- ❖ Place the chicken breasts in airtight containers or Ziploc bags; keep in your refrigerator for 3 to 4 days.
- ❖ For freezing, place the chicken breasts in airtight containers or heavy-duty freezer bags. It will maintain the best quality for about 4 months. Defrost in the refrigerator.
- ❖ Store dressing in your refrigerator for 3 to 4 days. Dress the salad and garnish with fresh avocado. Bon appétit!

264) EASY TO COOK RIBS

	Cooking Time: 8 Hours	Servings: 4

- ✓ 1 pound baby back ribs
- ✓ 4 tbsp coconut aminos
- ✓ 1/4 cup dry red wine
- ✓ 1/2 tsp cayenne pepper
- ✓ 1 garlic clove, crushed
- ✓ 1 tsp Italian herb mix
- ✓ 1 tbsp butter
- ✓ 1 tsp Serrano pepper, minced
- ✓ 1 Italian pepper, thinly sliced
- ✓ 1 tsp grated lemon zest

- ❖ Butter the sides and bottom of your Crock pot. Place the pork and peppers on the bottom.
- ❖ Add in the remaining ingredients.
- ❖ Slow cook for 9 hours on Low heat setting.
- ❖ Storing
- ❖ Divide the baby back ribs into four portions. Place each portion of the ribs along with the peppers in an airtight container; keep in your refrigerator for 3 to days.
- ❖ For freezing, place the ribs in airtight containers or heavy-duty freezer bags. Freeze up to 4 to months. Defrost in the refrigerator. Reheat in your oven at 250 degrees F until heated through.

265) CLASSIC BRIE-STUFFED MEATBALLS

	Cooking Time: 25 Minutes	Servings: 5

- ✓ 2 eggs, beaten
- ✓ 1 pound ground pork
- ✓ 1/3 cup double cream
- ✓ 1 tbsp fresh parsley
- ✓ Kosher salt and ground black pepper
- ✓ 1 tsp dried rosemary
- ✓ 10 (1-inch cubes of brie cheese
- ✓ 2 tbsp scallions, minced
- ✓ 2 cloves garlic, minced

- ❖ Mix all ingredients, except for the brie cheese, until everything is well incorporated.
- ❖ Roll the mixture into 10 patties; place a piece of cheese in the center of each patty and roll into a ball.
- ❖ Roast in the preheated oven at 0 degrees F for about 20 minutes.
- ❖ Storing
- ❖ Place the meatballs in airtight containers or Ziploc bags; keep in your refrigerator for up to 3 to 4 days.
- ❖ Freeze the meatballs in airtight containers or heavy-duty freezer bags. Freeze up to 3 to 4 months. To defrost, slowly reheat in a saucepan. Bon appétit!

Nutrition: 302 Calories; 13g Fat; 1.9g Carbs; 33.4g Protein; 0.3g Fiber

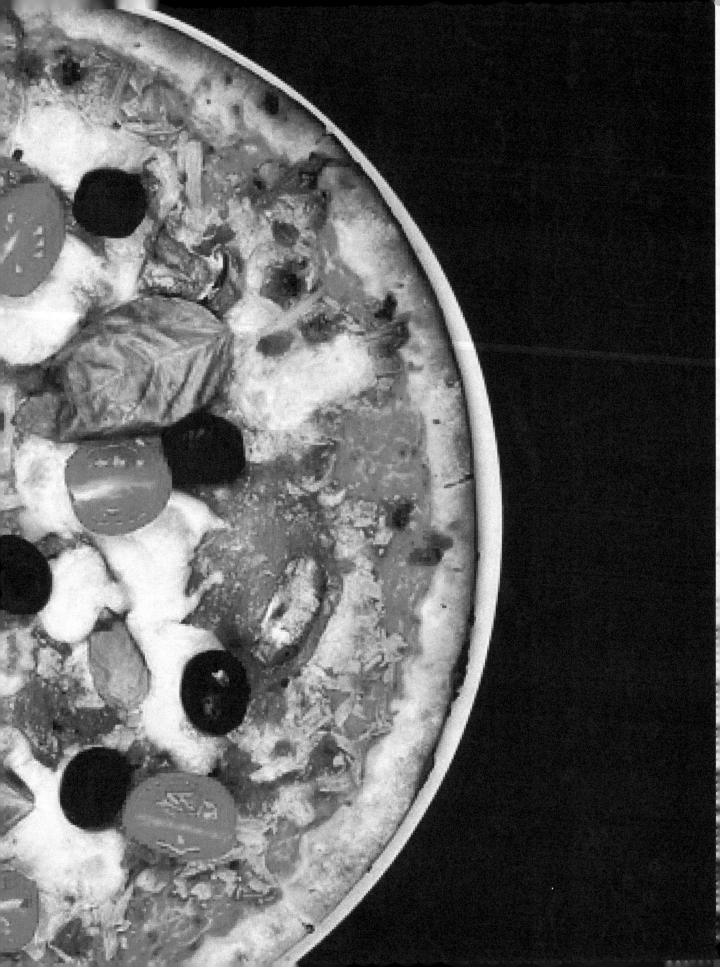

Chapter 4. THE BEST RECIPES

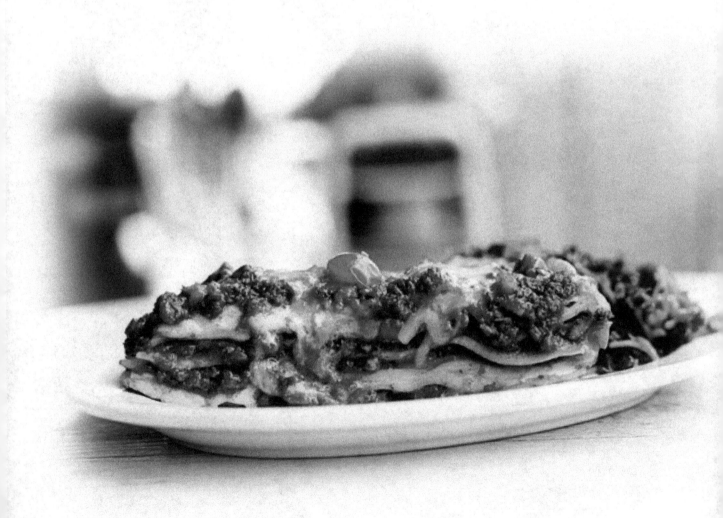

266) ITALIAN BAKED ZUCCHINI WITH THYME AND PARMESAN

Preparation Time: 10 minutes	Cooking Time: 20 minutes	Servings: 4

Ingredients:

- ✓ Four sliced zucchinis
- ✓ 1/2 tsp dried thyme
- ✓ 1/2 cup shredded Parmesan cheese
- ✓ 1/2 tsp dried oregano
- ✓ 2 tbsp olive oil
- ✓ 1/4 tsp garlic powder
- ✓ Kosher salt to taste
- ✓ 1/2 tsp dried basil
- ✓ Black pepper to taste
- ✓ 2 tbsp chopped parsley

Directions:

- ❖ Mix all the ingredients in a large bowl except zucchini.
- ❖ Make a layer of zucchini over a baking sheet sprayed with oil.
- ❖ Transfer the cheese mixture over zucchini and pour olive oil over them.
- ❖ Bake in a preheated oven at 350 degrees for 15 minutes, followed by broiling for three minutes.
- ❖ Serve and enjoy it.

267) ITALIAN BABA GANOUSH

Preparation Time: 10 minutes	Cooking Time: 40 minutes	Servings: 4

Ingredients:

- ✓ One eggplant
- ✓ 1 tbsp Greek yogurt
- ✓ olive oil
- ✓ 1.5 tbsp tahini paste
- ✓ 1 tbsp lime juice
- ✓ One garlic clove
- ✓ Salt to taste
- ✓ 1 tsp cayenne pepper
- ✓ Pepper to taste
- ✓ ½ tsp sumac for garnishing
- ✓ Parsley leaves for garnishing
- ✓ Toasted pine nuts for garnishing

Directions:

- ❖ Make slits in eggplant's skin.
- ❖ Place eggplant skin side upwards in a baking tray.
- ❖ Spray olive oil over eggplant.
- ❖ Bake in a preheated oven at 425 degrees for 40 minutes.
- ❖ Scoop the inner flesh of eggplant out and shift in a food processor. Add garlic, cayenne, yogurt, lime juice, salt, tahini, sumac, pepper, and blend. The baba ganoush is ready.
- ❖ You can refrigerator for better results for 60 minutes and sprinkle oil, sumac, parsley, and nuts and serve.

268) SICILIAN SALMON FISH STICKS

Preparation Time: 10 minutes	Cooking Time: 18 minutes	Servings: 4

- ✓ Fish Sticks
- ✓ 2 lb salmon fillet
- ✓ 1/4 tsp salt
- ✓ 1/4 tsp black pepper
- ✓ First coating
- ✓ 1/2 tsp garlic powder
- ✓ 1/2 tsp dried thyme
- ✓ 1 cup almond meal
- ✓ 1/2 tsp sea salt
- ✓ 1/4 tsp black pepper
- ✓ Second coating
- ✓ 1/2 tsp salt
- ✓ 2/3 cup chickpea flour
- ✓ Third coating
- ✓ Two eggs
- ✓ Dipping Sauce
- ✓ 1/4 tsp salt
- ✓ 1/4 cup Greek yogurt
- ✓ 1 tsp lemon juice
- ✓ 1 tbsp Dijon mustard
- ✓ 1/2 tsp dill
- ✓ 1/8 tsp garlic powder

Directions:

- ❖ Whisk all the ingredients for the dipping sauce list in a bowl and set aside. The dipping sauce is ready.
- ❖ Mix garlic, thyme, and almond meal in a bowl. The first coating is ready.
- ❖ Add chickpea flour in another bowl. The second coating is ready.
- ❖ Beat the eggs in another bowl. Set aside.
- ❖ Sprinkle pepper and salt over sliced fish with removed skin.
- ❖ First, coat the fish with chickpea flour, followed by coating with egg and almond meal coating.
- ❖ Aline coated fish pieces in a baking sheet covered with parchment paper.
- ❖ Bake in a preheated oven at 400 degrees for 18 minutes.
- ❖ Serve baked fish with dipping sauce and serve.

Nutrition: Calories: 92 kcal Fat: 5.7 g Protein: 14.4 g Carbs: 4.5 g Fiber: 1.3 g

269) AFRICAN BAKED FALAFEL

Preparation Time: 10 minutes	Cooking Time: 24 minutes	Servings: 15 patties

Ingredients:

- ✓ 15 oz chickpeas
- ✓ Three cloves garlic
- ✓ 1/4 cup chopped onion
- ✓ 1/2 cup parsley
- ✓ 2 tsp lemon juice
- ✓ 1/2 tsp baking soda
- ✓ 1 tbsp olive oil
- ✓ 1 tsp ground cumin
- ✓ 3/4 tsp salt
- ✓ 1 tsp coriander
- ✓ One pinch of cayenne
- ✓ 3 tbsp oat flour

Directions:

- ❖ Blend all the ingredients except oat flour and baking soda in a food processor to get roughly a blended mixture.
- ❖ Transfer the mixture to a bowl and add oat flour and baking soda. Using hands, mix the dough well.
- ❖ Make patties out of the falafel mixture and set aside for 15 minutes.
- ❖ Bake the falafel patties in a preheated oven at 375 degrees for 12 minutes and serve.

Nutrition: Calories: 143 kcal Fat: 5 g Protein: 6 g Carbs: 24 g Fiber: 6 g

270) GREEK CHIA YOGURT PUDDING

Preparation Time: 10 minutes	Cooking Time: 0 minute	Servings: 4

Ingredients:

- ✓ 3/4 cup milk
- ✓ 11 oz f Vanilla Yogurt
- ✓ 2 tbsp pure maple syrup
- ✓ 1 tsp vanilla extract
- ✓ 1/8 tsp salt
- ✓ 1/4 cup chia seeds
- ✓ Sliced almonds for garnishing

Directions:

- ❖ Whisk all the ingredients in a large bowl. Set aside for 24 hours in the refrigerator.
- ❖ Mix the mixture gently after 24 hours and serve after garnishing.

Nutrition: Calories: 179 kcal Fat: 5.6 g Protein: 10.1 g Carbs: 22.3 g Fiber: 6 g

271) EASY ITALIAN-STYLE FARFALLE

Preparation Time: 10 minutes	Cooking Time: 15 minutes	Servings: 7

Ingredients:

- ✓ 12 oz farfalle pasta
- ✓ ½ cup olive oil
- ✓ ¼ cup chopped basil leaves
- ✓ 1 lb crumbled chorizo sausage
- ✓ ½ cup pine nuts
- ✓ ½ cup shredded parmesan cheese
- ✓ Two chopped garlic cloves
- ✓ 1 cup diced tomato
- ✓ ¼ cup red wine vinegar

Directions:

- ❖ In a saucepan, boil water with added salt.
- ❖ Add pasta and cook until pasta is done.
- ❖ In a pan, cook chorizo over medium flame. Stir in nuts and cook for five minutes.
- ❖ Mix garlic and cook for a minute before removing the pan from the flame.
- ❖ Transfer cooked pasta, vinegar, cheese, cooked chorizo mixture, olive oil, tomatoes, and basil. Mix well to coat everything and serve.

Nutrition: Calories: 692 kcal Fat: 48 g Protein: 26.9 g Carbs: 39.7 g Fiber: 15 g

272) SPECIAL POTATO WEDGES

Preparation Time: 5 minutes	Cooking Time: 30 minutes	Servings: 4

Ingredients:

- ✓ Two wedges cut potatoes
- ✓ ½ tsp salt
- ✓ ½ tsp paprika
- ✓ 1.5 tbsp olive oil
- ✓ ½ tsp chili powder
- ✓ 1/8 black pepper

Directions:

- ❖ Combine all the ingredients in a bowl.
- ❖ Transfer the mixture to an air fryer basket and cook in a preheated air fryer at 400 degrees for eight minutes from both sides.
- ❖ Serve and enjoy it.

273) ORIGINAL GREEK-STYLE POTATOES

Preparation Time: 20 minutes	Cooking Time: 120 minutes	Servings: 4

Ingredients:

- ✓ 1/3 cup olive oil
- ✓ Two chopped garlic cloves
- ✓ 1.5 cups water
- ✓ Black pepper to taste
- ✓ ¼ cup lemon juice
- ✓ 1 tsp rosemary
- ✓ 1 tsp thyme
- ✓ Two chicken bouillon cubes
- ✓ Six chopped potatoes

Directions:

- ❖ Mix all the ingredients in a large bowl and pour over the potatoes placed in the baking tray.
- ❖ Bake in a preheated oven at 350 degrees for 90 minutes.
- ❖ Serve and enjoy it.

274) ORGINIAL ITALIAN-STYLE CHICKEN WRAP

Preparation Time: 10 minutes	Cooking Time: 20 minutes	Servings: 4

Ingredients:

- ✓ 2 tbsp butter
- ✓ 1/2 cup mayonnaise
- ✓ 1/2 lb boneless chicken breasts
- ✓ 1/4 cup shredded Parmesan cheese
- ✓ 2 cups shredded romaine lettuce
- ✓ Four flour tortillas
- ✓ Two sliced Roma tomatoes
- ✓ 1/2 cup crushed croutons
- ✓ 16 basil leaves

Directions:

- ❖ Cook chicken over medium flame in melted butter for 20 minutes.
- ❖ Slice the chicken into strips.
- ❖ Whisk cheese and mayonnaise and pour over the tortilla.
- ❖ Place lettuce followed by chicken, basil, tomato, and croutons on tortilla and wrap.
- ❖ Serve and enjoy it.

275) Lovely Avocado Caprese wrap

Preparation Time: 20 minutes	Cooking Time: 0 minute	Servings: 3

✓ Two tortillas
✓ Balsamic vinegar as needed
✓ One ball mozzarella cheese grated
✓ 1/2 cup arugula leaves
✓ One sliced tomato

✓ 2 tbsp basil leaves
✓ Kosher salt to taste
✓ One sliced avocado
✓ Olive oil as required
✓ Black pepper to taste

Directions:

❖ Place tomato slices and cheese, followed by avocado and basil. Over one side of the tortilla.
❖ Pour olive oil and vinegar. Drizzle pepper and salt.
❖ Wrap the tortilla and serve.

276) DELICIOUS CHICKEN SALAD WITH AVOCADO AND GREEK YOGURT

Preparation Time: 10 minutes	Cooking Time: 0 minute	Servings: 4

Ingredients:

✓ 1 cup plain yogurt
✓ 1 tbsp lemon juice
✓ One mashed avocado
✓ 1/3 cup dried cranberries
✓ Kosher salt to taste
✓ 2 cups shredded chicken

✓ Black pepper to taste
✓ 3/4 cup chopped celery
✓ 1/3 cup chopped pecans
✓ 1/2 cup chopped red grapes
✓ 1/3 cup chopped red onion
✓ 2 tbsp chopped tarragon

Directions:

❖ Whisk all the ingredients in a large mixing bowl.
❖ Serve as a salad and enjoy it.

277) EASY CHICKEN SHAWARMA PITAS

Preparation Time: 10 minutes	Cooking Time: 30 minutes	Servings: 6

✓ ¾ tbsp cumin
✓ ¾ tbsp coriander
✓ ¾ tbsp turmeric powder
✓ One sliced onion
✓ ¾ tbsp garlic powder
✓ ½ tsp cloves
✓ ¾ tbsp paprika

✓ 1 tbsp lemon juice
✓ ½ tsp cayenne pepper
✓ Eight boneless chicken
✓ Salt to taste
✓ 1/3 cup olive oil
✓ Pita bread
✓ Tahini sauce

Directions:

❖ In a bowl, add sliced chicken pieces, onions, cumin, garlic, cloves, olive oil, turmeric, paprika, lemon juice, salt, and coriander. Toss well to coat chicken evenly. Set aside for three hours in the refrigerator.
❖ Transfer the chicken pieces along with the marinade in a baking tray sprayed with oil.
❖ Bake in a preheated oven at 425 degrees for 30 minutes.
❖ Spread tahini sauce in pita bread and add baked chicken pieces. You can also add your favorite salad.
❖ Serve and enjoy it.

278)   SIMPLE RED LENTIL SOUP

Preparation Time: 10 minutes	Cooking Time: 45 minutes	Servings: 4

		Directions:
✓ Four minced garlic cloves	✓ 4 cups vegetable broth	❖ Cook carrots and onions in ¼ cup of heated olive oil in a Dutch oven over medium flame for five minutes.
✓ ¼ cup olive oil	✓ 1 tsp salt	❖ Stir in thyme, cumin, garlic, and curry powder,
✓ 1 tsp curry powder	✓ 2 cups of water	❖ Cook for half a minute.
✓ Two chopped carrots	✓ One pinch of red pepper flakes	❖ Add tomatoes and cook for another five minutes.
✓ 2 tsp ground cumin	✓ 1 cup chopped kale	❖ Add pepper flakes, broth, salt, lentils, black pepper, and water in a Dutch oven.
✓ One chopped onion	✓ Black pepper to taste	❖ Let it boil. Cover the oven and lower the flame and let it simmer for 30 minutes.
✓ ½ tsp dried thyme	✓ 1.5 tbsp lemon juice	❖ Blend a portion of soup of about two cups in a food processor and transfer it into the pot again.
✓ 1 cup brown lentils		❖ Mix chopped greens and cook for another five minutes.
✓ 28 oz diced tomatoes		❖ Remove from the flame and mix lemon juice and serve.

Nutrition: Calories: 366 kcal Fat: 15.5 g Protein: 14.5 g Carbs: 47.8 g Fiber: 10.8 g

279)   EASY SALMON SOUP

Preparation Time: 10 minutes	Cooking Time: 12 minutes	Servings: 4

Ingredients:		Directions:
	✓ One sliced carrot	❖ Cook onions, garlic, and bell pepper in heated olive oil in a pot over medium flame for four minutes.
✓ Olive oil	✓ ¾ tsp coriander	❖ Stir in the dill and cook for half a minute.
✓ ½ chopped green bell pepper	✓ Kosher salt to taste	❖ Pour broth into the pot. Add carrot, potatoes, salt, spices, and pepper.
✓ Four chopped green onions	✓ ½ tsp cumin	❖ Let it boil. Reduce the flame and let it simmer for six minutes.
✓ Four minced garlic cloves	✓ Black pepper to taste	❖ Add salmon and cook for five more minutes.
✓ 5 cups chicken broth	✓ Zest of one lemon	❖ Add lemon juice and zest and cook for one minute.
✓ 1 oz chopped dill	✓ 1 lb sliced salmon fillet	❖ Serve the soup and enjoy it.
✓ 1 lb sliced gold potatoes	✓ 1 tbsp lemon juice	
✓ 1 tsp dry oregano		

280) RICH FALAFEL SANDWICHES

Preparation Time: 20 minutes	Cooking Time: 10 minutes	Servings: 4 sandwiches

Ingredients:

- ✓ 4 Pita Breads
- ✓ 1 cup arugula
- ✓ 1 tbsp lemon
- ✓ 1/2 cup tahini sauce
- ✓ 12 falafels
- ✓ One sliced red onion
- ✓ 1/2 cup tabbouleh salad
- ✓ Three sprigs mint

Directions:

- ❖ Spread tahini sauce followed by the addition of arugula and crushed falafels over pita bread.
- ❖ Add tabbouleh salad, mint, and onions over pita and drizzle lemon juice.
- ❖ Wrap the pita bread and serve.

281) EASY ROASTED TOMATO AND BASIL SOUP

Preparation Time: 10 minutes	Cooking Time: 50 minutes	Servings: 6

Ingredients:

- ✓ 3 lb halved Roma tomatoes
- ✓ Olive oil
- ✓ Two chopped carrots
- ✓ Salt to taste
- ✓ Two chopped yellow onions
- ✓ Black pepper to taste
- ✓ Five minced garlic cloves
- ✓ 2 oz basil leaves
- ✓ 1 cup crushed tomatoes
- ✓ Three thyme sprigs
- ✓ 1 tsp dry oregano
- ✓ 2 tsp thyme leaves
- ✓ ½ tsp paprika
- ✓ 2.5 cups water
- ✓ ½ tsp cumin
- ✓ 1 tbsp lime juice

Directions:

- ❖ Mix salt, olive oil, carrot, black pepper, and tomatoes in a bowl.
- ❖ Transfer carrot mixture to a baking tray and bake in a preheated oven at 450 degrees for 30 minutes.
- ❖ Blend baked tomato mixture in a blender. You can use a little water if needed during blending.
- ❖ Sauté onions in heated olive oil over medium flame in a pot for three minutes.
- ❖ Mix garlic and cook for one more minute.
- ❖ Transfer the blended tomato mixture to the pot, followed by the addition of crushed tomatoes, water, spices, thyme, salt, basil, and pepper.
- ❖ Let it boil. Reduce the flame and simmer for 20 minutes.
- ❖ Drizzle lemon juice and serve.

282) GREEK-STYLE BLACK-EYED PEAS STEW

Preparation Time: 5 minutes	Cooking Time: 55 minutes	Servings: 6

Ingredients:

- ✓ Olive oil
- ✓ Four chopped garlic cloves
- ✓ 30 oz black-eyed peas
- ✓ One chopped yellow onion
- ✓ One chopped green bell pepper
- ✓ 15 oz diced tomato
- ✓ Three chopped carrots
- ✓ 1.5 tsp cumin
- ✓ One dry bay leaf
- ✓ 1 tsp dry oregano
- ✓ Kosher salt to taste
- ✓ ½ tsp red pepper flakes
- ✓ ½ tsp paprika
- ✓ Black pepper to taste
- ✓ 1 cup chopped parsley
- ✓ 1 tbsp of lime juice
- ✓ 2 cups of water

Directions:

- ❖ Cook garlic and onions in a heated oven in a Dutch oven over medium flame for five minutes with constant stirring.
- ❖ Stir in tomatoes, pepper, water, spices, bay leaf, and salt.
- ❖ Let it boil.
- ❖ Mix black-eyed beans and cook for five more minutes.
- ❖ Cover the oven and reduce the flame. Simmer for 30 minutes.
- ❖ Squeeze lemon juice and mix.
- ❖ Serve and enjoy.

283) GREEK CHICKEN GYROS WITH TZATZIKI SAUCE

Preparation Time: 10 minutes	Cooking Time: 8 minutes	Servings: 4

Ingredients:

- ✓ Greek Chicken
- ✓ 1 tbsp lemon juice
- ✓ 1/2 cup plain yogurt
- ✓ 1.25 tsp Italian-spiced salt
- ✓ 2 tbsp extra-virgin olive oil
- ✓ 1 cup Tzatziki sauce
- ✓ Four slices of pita bread
- ✓ Four chopped tomatoes
- ✓ 1/4 sliced red onion
- ✓ Tzatziki Sauce
- ✓ ½ halved cucumber
- ✓ ¾ cup Greek yogurt
- ✓ Two minced garlic cloves
- ✓ 1 tbsp red wine vinegar
- ✓ 1 tbsp chopped dill
- ✓ One pinch of kosher salt
- ✓ One pinch of black pepper

Directions:

- ❖ Marinate the chicken by mixing it with lemon juice, salt, and yogurt. Set aside for one hour.
- ❖ Heat olive oil in a skillet over medium flame.
- ❖ Add chicken without marinade and cook for five minutes from both sides. Transfer the cooked brown chicken to the plate.
- ❖ Mix all the ingredients of Tzatziki sauce in a bowl and set aside. The Tzatziki sauce is ready.
- ❖ Toast pita bread and place Tzatziki sauce, tomatoes, onions, and chicken pieces over pita bread. Wrap and serve.

Nutrition: Calories: 411 kcal Fat: 21 g Protein: 44 g Carbs: 10 g Fiber: 1 g

123

284) GREEK-STYLE CHICKEN MARINADE

Preparation Time: 5 minutes	Cooking Time: 15 minutes	Servings: 4

Ingredients:

- ✓ 1 lb boneless chicken breasts
- ✓ ¼ cup olive oil
- ✓ ½ tsp black pepper
- ✓ 1/3 cup Greek yogurt
- ✓ Four lemons
- ✓ 2 tbsp dried oregano
- ✓ Five minced garlic cloves
- ✓ 1 tsp kosher salt

Directions:

- ❖ Mix all the ingredients in a bowl and set aside for three hours.
- ❖ Preheat the grill and grill chicken and lemon slices for 20 minutes from both sides.
- ❖ Slice the grilled chicken and serve.

Nutrition: Calories: 304 kcal Fat: 19 g Protein: 25 g Carbs: 14 g Fiber: 4 g

285) ITALIAN STYLE CHICKEN QUINOA BOWL WITH BROCCOLI AND TOMATO

Preparation Time: 10 minutes	Cooking Time: 30 minutes	Servings: 3

Ingredients:

- ✓ Chicken
- ✓ 6 oz boneless chicken breast
- ✓ 1 cup Easy Roasted Feta and Broccoli
- ✓ 1/2 cup olive oil
- ✓ 1/2 tsp kosher salt
- ✓ Zest of one lemon
- ✓ 2 tsp dried oregano
- ✓ 1.5 tbsp lemon juice
- ✓ 1/4 tsp black pepper
- ✓ Two minced garlic cloves
- ✓ 1/2 cup Easy Roasted Tomatoes
- ✓ Quinoa
- ✓ 1 tsp kosher salt
- ✓ 1 cup dried quinoa
- ✓ Feta cheese to taste

Directions:

- ❖ Mix lemon juice, oregano, salt, olive oil, garlic, lemon zest, and pepper in a bowl.
- ❖ Add chicken and toss well. Set aside for one hour.
- ❖ Cook chicken in heat olive oil over medium flame for 15 minutes.
- ❖ Lower the flame and stir in tomatoes and broccoli and cook. Set aside.
- ❖ Add water and salt to a pot and bring it to a boil.
- ❖ Add quinoa and cook for ten minutes.
- ❖ Drain the quinoa and set aside.
- ❖ Add quinoa in a bowl, followed by the addition of chicken and veggies. Sprinkle salt, cheese, oil, and pepper.
- ❖ Serve and enjoy it.

Nutrition: Calories: 481 kcal Fat: 23 g Protein: 24 g Carbs: 45 g Fiber: 7 g

286) EASY CHICKEN PICCATA

Preparation Time: 10 minutes	Cooking Time: 10 minutes	Servings: 4

Ingredients:

- ✓ 1.5 lb boneless chicken breasts
- ✓ One lemon
- ✓ 2 tbsp canola oil
- ✓ 1 tsp kosher salt
- ✓ 1 cup chicken broth
- ✓ 1 tsp black pepper
- ✓ 2 tbsp capers
- ✓ 3 tbsp butter
- ✓ 1/3 cup all-purpose flour

Directions:

- ❖ Mix salt, flour, and pepper in a bowl. Coat chicken with the flour mixture. Set aside.
- ❖ Cook chicken pieces in heated butter and canola oil over medium flame for five minutes from both sides. Shift cooked pieces onto the plate.
- ❖ Lower the flame and pour broth and add sliced lemon, butter (1 tbsp), lemon juice, capers, and cook for five minutes.
- ❖ Pour the sauce over chicken pieces and serve with cauliflower or noodles.

Nutrition: Calories: 381 kcal Fat: 20 g Protein: 37 g Carbs: 11 g Fiber: 1 g

287) ITALIAN CHOPPED GRILLED VEGETABLE WITH FARRO

Preparation Time: 5 minutes	Cooking Time: 50 minutes	Servings: 2

Ingredients:

- 1 cup dried farro
- 1 Portobello mushroom
- 3 cups vegetable broth
- One sliced red bell pepper
- 1/2 sliced red onion
- 8 oz asparagus
- One sliced zucchini
- Olive oil as required
- 1/4 cup halved Kalamata olives
- One sliced yellow squash
- Kosher salt to taste
- 1-pint Greek yogurt
- Black pepper to taste
- 2 tbsp minced cucumber
- One chopped garlic clove
- 1 tbsp lemon juice
- 1 tsp chopped dill
- 1 tsp chopped mint
- Red bell pepper hummus
- 1/8 cup feta cheese

Directions:

- ❖ In a large pot, add broth and farro. Let it boil over a high flame.
- ❖ Lower the flame to medium and cook for half an hour with occasional stirring.
- ❖ Mix veggies with salt, olive oil, and pepper.
- ❖ Grill the veggies in a preheated grill until marks appear on them. Keep them aside.
- ❖ Whisk cucumber, salt, mint, dill, yogurt, lemon juice, and garlic in a bowl.
- ❖ Make the layers of farro, grilled veggies, hummus, olives, and cheese.
- ❖ Pour yogurt sauce and sprinkle mint and serve.

Nutrition: Calories: 140 kcal Fat: 6 g Protein: 4 g Carbs: 20 g Fiber: 5 g

288) QUICK PORK ESCALOPES IN 30 MINUTES WITH LEMONS AND CAPERS

Preparation Time: 10 minutes	Cooking Time: 20 minutes	Servings: 4

Ingredients:

- Four boneless pork chops
- 1/4 cup all-purpose flour
- Eight sage leaves
- kosher salt to taste
- 2 tbsp chopped parsley
- 4 tbsp butter
- Black pepper to taste
- 1 tbsp vegetable oil
- 1/4 cup capers
- 1/2 cup white wine
- 1 cup chicken stock
- One sliced lemon
- 4 tbsp lemon juice

Directions:

- ❖ One each pork chops, place two sage leaves on both sides. Set aside.
- ❖ In a bowl, whisk salt, flour, and pepper.
- ❖ Coat pork chops with flour. Keep the sage leaves in place.
- ❖ Melt butter in a skillet over medium flame.
- ❖ Cook pork chops for five minutes from both sides.
- ❖ Clean the skillet and melt butter in it.
- ❖ Pour wine and add capers in skillet. Cook to concentrate the wine.
- ❖ Pour stock, lemon slices, and lemon juice. Let it boil for five more minutes.
- ❖ Place pork in sauce and cook for two minutes.
- ❖ Sprinkle parsley and serve.

Nutrition: Calories: 415 kcal Fat: 7 g Protein: 31 g Carbs: 14 g Fiber: 8 g

289) GREEK-STYLE CHICKEN KEBABS

Preparation Time: 40 minutes	**Cooking Time:** 15 minutes	**Servings: 6**

Ingredients:

- ✓ 1 lb boneless chicken breasts
- ✓ 1/4 cup olive oil
- ✓ One sliced red bell pepper
- ✓ 1/3 cup Greek yogurt
- ✓ 10 tbsp lemons juice
- ✓ Four chopped garlic cloves
- ✓ Zest of one lemon
- ✓ 2 tbsp dried oregano
- ✓ 1/2 tsp black pepper
- ✓ One sliced zucchini
- ✓ 1 tsp kosher salt
- ✓ One sliced red onion

Directions:

- ❖ Whisk all the ingredients except chicken in a bowl. Add chicken and toss to coat chicken evenly. Set aside four hours for better results.
- ❖ Thread chicken, zucchini, onion, and bell pepper on the skewers.
- ❖ Grill the chicken, skewers on a preheated grill for 15 minutes, occasionally turning and basting with marinade.

Nutrition: Calories: 224 kcal Fat: 13 g Protein: 18 g Carbs: 13 g Fiber: 4 g

290) EASY PASTA WITH SHRIMP AND ROASTED RED PEPPERS AND ARTICHOKES

Preparation Time: 10 minutes	**Cooking Time:** 25 minutes	**Servings: 8**

Ingredients:

- ✓ 12 oz farfalle pasta
- ✓ 1/4 cup butter
- ✓ 1.5 lb shrimp
- ✓ Three chopped garlic cloves
- ✓ 1 cup sliced artichoke hearts
- ✓ 12 oz roasted and chopped red bell peppers
- ✓ 1/2 cup dry white wine
- ✓ 1/4 cup basil
- ✓ 1/2 cup whipping cream
- ✓ 3 tbsp drained capers
- ✓ 1 tsp grated lemon peel
- ✓ 3/4 cup feta cheese
- ✓ 2 tbsp lemon juice
- ✓ 2 oz toasted pine nuts

Directions:

- ❖ Boil water in a pot and cook pasta in it.
- ❖ Drain pasta and set aside.
- ❖ Melt butter in a skillet over medium flame. Sauté garlic and cook for one minute.
- ❖ Stir in shrimps and cook for about two minutes.
- ❖ Mix artichokes, capers, bell pepper, and wine. Let it boil.
- ❖ Lower the flame and let it simmer for two minutes with occasional stirring.
- ❖ Add whipping cream, lemon juice, and lemon zest.
- ❖ Let it boil for five minutes.
- ❖ Transfer the cooked shrimps over pasta and mix well.
- ❖ Spread cheese, basil, and nuts and serve.

Nutrition: Calories: 627 kcal Fat: 24 g Protein: 38 g Carbs: 58 g Fiber: 3 g

291)   CHICKEN CAPRESE QUICK IN 30 MINUTES

Preparation Time: 10 minutes	Cooking Time: 20 minutes	Servings: 4

Ingredients:

- ✓ Two boneless chicken breasts
- ✓ Black pepper to taste
- ✓ 1 tbsp butter
- ✓ 1 tbsp extra virgin olive oil
- ✓ 6 oz Pesto
- ✓ Eight chopped tomatoes
- ✓ Six grated mozzarella cheese
- ✓ Balsamic glaze as needed
- ✓ Kosher salt to taste
- ✓ Basil as required

Directions:

- ❖ Mix salt, sliced chicken, and pepper in a bowl. Set aside for ten minutes.
- ❖ Melt butter in a skillet over medium flame.
- ❖ Cook chicken pieces in melted butter for five minutes from both sides.
- ❖ Remove from the flame. Sprinkle pesto and place mozzarella cheese and tomatoes over chicken pieces.
- ❖ Bake in a preheated oven at 400 degrees for 12 minutes.
- ❖ Garnish with balsamic glaze and serve.

Nutrition: Calories: 232 kcal Fat: 15 g Protein: 18 g Carbs: 5 g Fiber: 1 g

292)   SPECIAL GRILLED LEMON CHICKEN SKEWERS

Preparation Time: 10 minutes	Cooking Time: 10 minutes	Servings: 6

Ingredients:

- ✓ Two boneless chicken breasts
- ✓ Seven green onions
- ✓ Four minced garlic cloves
- ✓ Three lemons
- ✓ 1 tbsp dried oregano
- ✓ 1 tsp kosher salt
- ✓ 1/4 cup olive oil
- ✓ 1/2 tsp black pepper

Directions:

- ❖ Whisk salt, lemon juice, olive oil, garlic, lemon zest, black pepper, oregano, and sliced chicken pieces in a bowl. Set aside for four hours.
- ❖ Thread chicken, onions, and lemon slices onto the skewer.
- ❖ Grill chicken skewers for 15 minutes on preheated grill over medium flames with often turning.
- ❖ Serve when chicken is fully cooked.

293)   TASTY JUICY SALMON BURGERS

Preparation Time: 10 minutes	Cooking Time: 4 minutes	Servings: 4

- ✓ 1.5 lb sliced salmon fillet
- ✓ 3 tbsp minced green onions
- ✓ 1 tsp coriander
- ✓ 2 tsp Dijon mustard
- ✓ 1/3 cup bread crumbs
- ✓ 1 tsp sumac
- ✓ 1 cup chopped parsley
- ✓ ½ tsp sweet paprika
- ✓ Kosher Salt to taste
- ✓ ¼ cup olive oil
- ✓ ½ tsp black pepper
- ✓ One lemon
- ✓ Toppings
- ✓ One sliced red onion
- ✓ Tzatziki Sauce
- ✓ One sliced tomato
- ✓ 6 oz baby arugula

Directions:

- ❖ Blend mustard and salmon in a blender.
- ❖ Shift the mixture in a container. Add all the spices, parsley, salt, and onions. Mix well and set aside for 30 minutes.
- ❖ Make patties out of salmon mixture and place in a tray.
- ❖ Coat all the patties with bread crumbs from both sides.
- ❖ Fry the patties in heated olive oil over medium flame for five minutes each from both sides.
- ❖ Drizzle lemon juice over the cooked patties.
- ❖ Spread Tzatziki sauce over the bun, followed by the layer of salmon, arugula, onions, and tomatoes. The salmon burgers are ready. Serve and enjoy it.

294) SPECIAL BRAISED EGGPLANT AND CHICKPEAS

Preparation Time: 20 minutes	Cooking Time: 55 minutes	Servings: 6

Ingredients		Directions
✓ 1.5 lb chopped eggplant ✓ Olive Oil ✓ Kosher salt ✓ One chopped yellow onion ✓ One chopped carrot ✓ One diced green bell pepper ✓ Six minced garlic cloves ✓ 1.5 tsp sweet paprika	✓ Two dry bay leaves ✓ 1 tsp organic coriander ✓ ¾ tsp cinnamon ✓ 1 tsp dry oregano ✓ ½ tsp organic turmeric ✓ 28 oz chopped tomato ✓ ½ tsp black pepper ✓ 30 oz chickpeas ✓ Handful parsley and mint for garnishing	❖ Sauté onions, carrots, and bell peppers in heated olive oil over medium flame for four minutes with constant stirring. ❖ Stir in salt, bay leaf, garlic, and spices and cook for one minute. ❖ Mix eggplant, chickpeas, tomato, and chickpea liquid. ❖ Let it boil for ten minutes. ❖ Remove the pan from flame and cover. ❖ Now, bake in a preheated oven at 400 degrees for 45 minutes. ❖ Sprinkle herbs and serve with any sauce.

295) ITALIAN STYLE TUNA SALAD SANDWICHES

Preparation Time: 5 minutes	Cooking Time: 0 minute	Servings: 4

Ingredients		Directions
✓ 4 tsp red wine vinegar ✓ 4 tsp olive oil ✓ Eight bread slices ✓ ¼ cup chopped red onion ✓ 1/3 cup chopped sun-dried tomatoes	✓ ¼ tsp black pepper ✓ ¼ cup sliced olives ✓ 3 tbsp mayonnaise ✓ 2 tsp capers ✓ Four lettuce leaves ✓ 12 oz tuna	❖ Mix wine and olive oil. ❖ Brush bread from both sides with oil mixture. ❖ Mix all the ingredients except lettuce and bread slices in a bowl. ❖ Place lettuce on each bread slices brushed with oil. Spread tuna mixture and cover with second bread piece and serve.

296) MOROCCAN-STYLE VEGETABLE TAGINE

Preparation Time: 15 minutes	Cooking Time: 40 minutes	Servings: 5

Ingredients:		Directions:
✓ ¼ cup extra virgin olive oil ✓ Ten chopped garlic cloves ✓ Two chopped yellow onions ✓ Two chopped carrots ✓ One sliced sweet potato ✓ Two sliced potatoes ✓ Salt ✓ 1 tsp coriander	✓ 1 tbsp Harissa spice ✓ 1 tsp cinnamon ✓ 2 cups tomatoes ✓ ½ tsp turmeric ✓ ½ cup chopped dried apricot ✓ 2 cups cooked chickpeas ✓ Handful fresh parsley leaves ✓ ½ cup vegetable broth ✓ 1 tbsp lemon juice	❖ Sauté onions in heated olive oil at high flame for five minutes in a Dutch oven. ❖ Stir in veggies, salt, garlic, and spices. Mix well and cook for eight minutes over medium flame with constant stirring. ❖ Mix in broth, apricot, and tomatoes and cook for the next ten minutes. ❖ Reduce the flame and let it simmer for 25 minutes. ❖ Add chickpeas and cook for five minutes. ❖ Sprinkle parsley and lemon juice and mix well. ❖ Serve and enjoy it.

297)	ITALIAN-STYLE GRILLED BALSAMIC CHICKEN WITH OLIVE TAPENADE	
Preparation Time: 10 minutes	**Cooking Time:** 30 minutes	**Servings:** 2

Ingredients:

- ✓ Two boneless chicken breasts
- ✓ 1/4 cup olive oil
- ✓ 1/4 cup balsamic vinegar
- ✓ 1/8 cup garlic mustard
- ✓ 1.5 tbsp balsamic vinegar
- ✓ Three minced garlic cloves
- ✓ 1 tbsp lemon juice
- ✓ 1 tbsp chopped herbs of choice
- ✓ 1 tsp kosher salt
- ✓ 1/2 tsp black pepper

Directions:

- ❖ Combine garlic, balsamic vinegar, lemon juice, pepper, olive oil, herbs, salt, and mustard in a bowl. Add chicken and toss well to coat chicken.
- ❖ Set aside for three hours.
- ❖ Brush oil over chicken pieces and grill gates.
- ❖ Cook chicken on grill gates for ten minutes from both sides.
- ❖ Occasionally brush the chicken with marinade while grilling it.
- ❖ When marks appear over the chicken, shift the chicken to the grill gate's cooler side and cook there for 12 minutes.
- ❖ Again, shift the chicken to the heated side of the grill gate and cook for ten more minutes.
- ❖ Place the grilled chicken on a plate and cover to keep it warm.
- ❖ Serve and enjoy it.

Nutrition: Calories: 352 kcal Fat: 21 g Protein: 35 mg Carbs: 5 g Fiber: 1 g

298)	ITALIAN LINGUINE AND ZUCCHINI NOODLES WITH SHRIMP	
Preparation Time: 20 minutes	**Cooking Time:** 20 minutes	**Servings:** 6

Ingredients:

- ✓ 2/3 cup extra virgin olive oil
- ✓ 1 lb shrimp
- ✓ Four minced garlic cloves
- ✓ Black pepper to taste
- ✓ 12 oz wheat linguine
- ✓ kosher salt to taste
- ✓ 3 tbsp butter
- ✓ Three zucchinis
- ✓ One lemon zested
- ✓ 1 tsp red chili flakes
- ✓ 3 tbsp lemon juice
- ✓ A handful of chopped parsley
- ✓ 1/2 cup shredded Parmesan cheese

Directions:

- ❖ Add salt, garlic, shrimps, pepper, and olive oil. Toss well to coat evenly. Keep it aside.
- ❖ Pour water into a pot and add salt to it. Let it boil and cook linguine in boiling water. Drain linguine and set aside.
- ❖ Heat olive oil in a skillet over medium heat and cook shrimps in it for three minutes from both sides. Shift the cooked shrimps into the plate.
- ❖ Melt butter in the same pan and sauté garlic, lemon juice, chili flakes, and lemon zest for one minute.
- ❖ Pour in pasta water in another pan and cook for three minutes. Add zucchini noodles and cook for two minutes with constant stirring.
- ❖ Transfer the noodles to the garlic mixture pan. Add linguine and cheese. Toss well.
- ❖ Pour in more of the pasta water to make a sauce of the desired level.
- ❖ Add shrimp, zucchini, salt, and pepper, and mix well.
- ❖ You can spread more cheese if you like.
- ❖ Garnish with parsley and serve.

Nutrition: Calories: 521 kcal Fat: 22 g Protein: 28 g Carbs: 52 g Fiber: 4 g

299) NAPOLI CAPRESE AVOCADO TOAST

Preparation Time:	Cooking Time: 10 minutes	Servings: 1

Ingredients:

- ✓ Two avocados
- ✓ ¼ cup chopped basil leaves
- ✓ 2 tsp lemon juice
- ✓ 4 oz sliced mozzarella
- ✓ Sea salt to taste
- ✓ Four toasted slices of bread
- ✓ Black pepper to taste
- ✓ 1 cup halved grape tomatoes
- ✓ Balsamic glaze for drizzling

Directions:

- ❖ In a bowl, add sliced avocados, salt, lemon juice, and pepper and mix well.
- ❖ Over medium flame, lightly toast the bread.
- ❖ Using a knife, spread avocados mixture over bread slices.
- ❖ Sprinkle salt, basil, cheese, pepper, balsamic glaze, and tomatoes.
- ❖ Serve and enjoy it.

300) SPECIAL OMELETTE OF ASPARAGUS AND MUSHROOMS WITH GOAT CHEESE

Preparation Time:	Cooking Time: 8 minutes	Servings: 4

Ingredients:

- ✓ 2 tbsp goat cheese
- ✓ Two eggs
- ✓ 1 pinch of kosher salt
- ✓ 1 tsp of milk
- ✓ 1 tbsp butter
- ✓ Five trimmed asparagus spears
- ✓ Three sliced brown mushrooms
- ✓ 1 tbsp chopped green onion

Directions:

- ❖ In a pan, cook mushrooms over medium flame for about three minutes.
- ❖ Stir in asparagus and cook for two more minutes.
- ❖ In a bowl, add one tsp of water, eggs, and salt and mix well.
- ❖ Add the egg mixture to the mushroom mixture, followed by a drizzling of goat cheese and green onions.
- ❖ Let them cook well until the egg mixture is properly formed.
- ❖ Shift the pan to the preheated oven and bake for three minutes.
- ❖ Drizzle cheese and serve.

Nutrition: Calories: 331 kcal Fat: 26 g Protein: 20 g Carbs: 7 g Fiber: 2 g

301) ITALIAN STYLE STRATA

Preparation Time: 20 minutes	Cooking Time: 55 minutes	Servings: 7

Ingredients:

- ✓ 2 tbsp olive oil
- ✓ One minced clove garlic
- ✓ 1/2 diced yellow onion
- ✓ 1 lb chicken sausage
- ✓ 1/2 cup halved Kalamata olives
- ✓ 6 cups white bread
- ✓ 1/2 cup chopped sun-dried tomatoes
- ✓ 1/4 cup chopped fresh basil
- ✓ 1/2 cup crumbled feta cheese
- ✓ Eight eggs
- ✓ Salt and pepper to taste
- ✓ 2 cups of milk
- ✓ Red pepper flakes

Directions:

- ❖ Heat butter and oil over medium flame in skillet. Sauté onions for two minutes. Stir in garlic and chicken sausage.
- ❖ Cook until sausages are done.
- ❖ Mix olives, cook sausages, onions, sun-dried tomatoes, pepper, bread, garlic, feta cheese, basil, red chili flakes, and salt.
- ❖ Mix milk and egg in a small bowl and add in sausage mixture.
- ❖ Pour the sausage mixture into the baking tray.
- ❖ Bake in preheated oven for 50 minutes and serve after garnishing with basil.

Nutrition: Calories: 297 kcal Fat: 9.5 g Protein: 17.9 g Carbs: 36 g Fiber: 3.1 g

302) ITALIAN STYLE SLOW COOKER EGG CASSEROLE

Preparation Time: 25 minutes	Cooking Time: 480 minutes	Servings: 10

✓ 2 oz cut prosciutto ✓ 3 cups sliced cremini mushrooms ✓ 1 tbsp butter ✓ 1/2 chopped red pepper ✓ 10 oz chopped spinach ✓ 16 oz ORE-IDA Diced Hash Brown Potatoes	✓ 1 cup sliced artichoke hearts ✓ 8 oz cheddar & Swiss Cheese ✓ 1/4 cup chopped sun-dried tomato ✓ 4 oz goat cheese ✓ 1 tbsp Dijon Mustard ✓ Eight eggs ✓ fresh basil leaves for garnish ✓ 2 cups whole milk	❖ Sauté prosciutto for four minutes in a pan over medium flame. Set aside. ❖ In the same pan, cook bell pepper and mushrooms in the melted butter. ❖ Make layers of potatoes, bell pepper and mushroom mixture, spinach, sundried tomatoes, artichoke hearts, Swiss and cheddar cheese, and goat cheese in the slow cooker. ❖ Mix mustard, milk, salt, eggs, and pepper spread over the veggie's layers in a slow cooker. ❖ Spread prosciutto over the top and cook for about ten minutes on low flame. ❖ Sprinkle basil and serve.

303) SPECIAL SHEET PAN EGGS AND VEGGIES

Preparation Time: 10 minutes	Cooking Time: 15 minutes	Servings: 6

✓ One sliced bell pepper (green, red, and orange) ✓ One sliced red onion ✓ Salt to taste ✓ Black pepper to taste ✓ 2 tsp za'atar blend, ✓ 1 tsp ground cumin and	✓ 1 tsp Aleppo chili pepper ✓ Extra virgin olive oil as required ✓ Six eggs ✓ A handful of Chopped fresh parsley ✓ One diced Roma tomato ✓ Crumbled feta cheese	❖ In a bowl, whisk bell peppers, onions, salt, zaatar, Aleppo chili, cumin, olive oil, and black pepper. Mix well. ❖ Shift the bell pepper mixture over the baking pan. ❖ Bake in a preheated oven at 400 degrees for 15 minutes. ❖ Make holes in baked vegetable mixture and crack one egg in each hole. ❖ Again, bake for eight minutes. ❖ Sprinkle cheese, parsley, and tomatoes and serve.

304) SPECIAL HUMMUS TOAST

Preparation Time: 10 minutes	Cooking Time: 0 minute	Servings: 4

✓ Hummus
✓ Whole-grain bread seeded
✓ Topping option 1
✓ Sprouts
✓ Sliced avocado
✓ Black sesame seeds
✓ Topping option 2

✓ Za'atar spice
✓ Roasted chickpeas
✓ Topping option 3
✓ Sunflower seeds
✓ Pumpkin seeds
✓ Hemp seeds
✓ Sesame seeds

Directions:

❖ Spread hummus using a knife over toast and top with any of the topping options given in ingredients and serve.

305) ORIGINAL BREAKFAST EGG MUFFINS

Preparation Time: 15 minutes	Cooking Time: 20 minutes	Servings: 6

Ingredients:

✓ Base
✓ Salt to taste
✓ 12 eggs
✓ 2 tbsp chopped onion
✓ Black pepper to taste
✓ Tomato spinach mozzarella
✓ Eight sliced cherry tomatoes
✓ 1/4 cup chopped spinach
✓ 1/4 cup grated mozzarella cheese

✓ Bacon cheddar
✓ 1/4 cup grated cheddar cheese
✓ 1/4 cup chopped bacon
✓ Garlic mushroom pepper
✓ 1/4 cup diced red capsicum
✓ 1/4 cup sliced brown mushrooms
✓ 1/4 tsp minced garlic powder
✓ 1 tbsp chopped parsley

Directions:

❖ Mix onions, salt, eggs, and black pepper in a bowl.
❖ Pour egg mixture in muffin cups greased with oil.
❖ Use all three toppings to top each of the muffin cups.
❖ Bake in a preheated oven at 350 degrees for twenty minutes.
❖ Serve and enjoy it.

Nutrition: Calories: 82 kcal Fat: 5 g Protein: 6 g Carbs: 1 g Fiber: 1 g

306) DELICIOUS FOUL MUDAMMAS

Preparation Time: 15 minutes	Cooking Time: 10 minutes	Servings: 5

Ingredients:

- ✓ Extra virgin olive oil
- ✓ Kosher salt to taste
- ✓ 30 oz plain fava beans
- ✓ 1 tsp ground cumin
- ✓ One lemon juice
- ✓ 1 cup chopped parsley
- ✓ Two chopped hot peppers
- ✓ One diced tomato
- ✓ Two chopped garlic cloves
- ✓ To serve
- ✓ Warm pit bread
- ✓ Green onions
- ✓ Sliced cucumbers
- ✓ Sliced tomatoes
- ✓ Olives

Directions:

- ❖ Pour half cup of water, salt, beans, and cumin in a pan over medium flame and cook.
- ❖ When beans are done, mash them using a masher.
- ❖ Lightly blend garlic, lemon juice, and hot peppers.
- ❖ Transfer roughly blended hot pepper mixture over mashed beans.
- ❖ Ass olive oil, parsley, hot pepper slices, and chopped tomatoes and serve with veggies or bread.

Nutrition: Calories: 142 kcal Fat: 1 g Protein: 10 g Carbs: 25 g Fiber: 10 g

307) TASTY TAHINI BANANA SHAKES

Preparation Time: 5 minutes	Cooking Time: 0 minute	Servings: 3

Ingredients:

- ✓ ¼ cup ice, crushed
- ✓ 1 ½ cups almond milk
- ✓ ¼ cup tahini
- ✓ 4 Medjool dates
- ✓ Two sliced bananas
- ✓ One pinch of ground cinnamon

Directions:

- ❖ Blend all the ingredients in the blender to obtain a creamy and smooth mixture.
- ❖ Pour mixture in cups and serve after sprinkling cinnamon over the top.

Nutrition: Calories: 299 kcal Fat: 12.4 g Protein: 5.7 g Carbs: 47.7 g Fiber: 5.6 g

308)   SIMPLE SHAKSHUKA

Preparation Time: 15 minutes	Cooking Time: 20 minutes	Servings: 6

Ingredients:

- ✓ 1 tsp ground cumin
- ✓ 2 tbsp olive oil
- ✓ One chopped red bell pepper
- ✓ Six eggs
- ✓ ¼ tsp salt
- ✓ Three minced cloves garlic
- ✓ Ground black pepper to taste
- ✓ 2 tbsp tomato paste
- ✓ ½ tsp smoked paprika
- ✓ ¼ tsp red pepper flakes
- ✓ 2 tbsp chopped cilantro for garnish
- ✓ ½ cup feta cheese
- ✓ One chopped yellow onion
- ✓ 28 oz fire-roasted tomatoes, crushed
- ✓ Crusty bread for serving

Directions:

- ❖ Heat oil in a skillet over medium flame and cook bell pepper, onions, and salt in it for six minutes with constant stirring.
- ❖ After six minutes, stir in tomato paste, red pepper flakes, cumin, garlic, and paprika. Cook for another two minutes.
- ❖ Add crushed tomatoes and cilantro to the onion mixture. Let it simmer.
- ❖ Reduce the flame and simmer for five minutes.
- ❖ Use salt and pepper to adjust the flavor.
- ❖ Crack eggs in small well made at different areas using a spoon. Pour tomato mixture over eggs to help them cook while staying intact.
- ❖ Bake the skillet in a preheated oven at 375 degrees for 12 minutes.
- ❖ Garnish with cilantro, flakes, and cheese and serve.

Nutrition: Calories: 216 kcal Fat: 12.8 g Protein: 11.2 g Carbs: 16.6 g Fiber: 4.4 g

309)   SPECIAL GREEN JUICE

Preparation Time: 15 minutes	Cooking Time: 0 minute	Servings: 2

Ingredients:

- ✓ 5 oz kale
- ✓ 1 tsp crushed ginger
- ✓ One apple
- ✓ Five trimmed celery stalks
- ✓ ½ English cucumber
- ✓ 1 oz parsley

Directions:

- ❖ Blend all the ingredients in the blender and pour into serving cups.

Nutrition: Calories: 92 kcal Fat: 0.8 g Protein: 2.8 g Carbs: 21 g Fiber: 6.2 g

310)   GREEK-STYLE CHICKEN GYRO SALAD

Preparation Time: 15 minutes	Cooking Time: 7 minutes	Servings: 4

Ingredients:

- ✓ Chicken
- ✓ 3 tsp dried oregano
- ✓ 2 tbsp olive oil
- ✓ 1 tbsp red wine vinegar
- ✓ 1.25 lb boneless chicken breasts
- ✓ 1 tsp ground black pepper
- ✓ 1 tbsp lemon juice
- ✓ 1 tsp Kosher salt
- ✓ Salad
- ✓ 1 cup diced English cucumber
- ✓ 6 cups lettuce
- ✓ 1 cup feta cheese diced
- ✓ 1 cup diced tomatoes
- ✓ 1/2 cup diced red onions
- ✓ 1 cup crushed pita chips
- ✓ Tzatziki Sauce
- ✓ 1 tbsp white wine vinegar
- ✓ 3/4 tsp Kosher salt
- ✓ 8 oz Greek yogurt
- ✓ One minced clove garlic
- ✓ 2/3 cup grated English cucumber
- ✓ 1 tbsp lemon juice
- ✓ 3/4 tsp ground black pepper
- ✓ 2 tsp dried dill weed
- ✓ One pinch of sugar

Directions:

- ❖ Heat oil in a skillet and add chicken, salt, oregano, and black pepper. Cook for five minutes over medium flame.
- ❖ Reduce the flame to low and add lemon juice and vinegar and simmer for five minutes.
- ❖ Continue cooking until the chicken is done. Now, the chicken is ready and set aside.
- ❖ Combine tomatoes, pita chips, chicken, lettuce, cucumber, and onions. Mix and set aside. The salad is ready.
- ❖ In another bowl, whisk yogurt, cucumber, garlic, lemon juice, vinegar, dill, salt, pepper, and sugar. Mix well. The sauce is ready.
- ❖ Now, pour the sauce over the salad and serve with cooked chicken.

Nutrition: Calories: 737 kcal Fat: 29 g Protein: 64 g Carbs: 54 g Fiber: 6 g

311)   TUSCAN-STYLE TUNA AND WHITE BEAN SALAD

Preparation Time: 5 minutes	Cooking Time: 0 minute	Servings: 2

Ingredients:

- ✓ 2 tbsp extra virgin olive oil
- ✓ 15 oz cannellini beans
- ✓ 4 cups spinach
- ✓ 5 oz white albacore
- ✓ 1/4 cup sliced olives
- ✓ 1/2 cup diced cherry tomatoes
- ✓ One sliced red onion
- ✓ 1/2 lemon
- ✓ Kosher salt to taste
- ✓ 1/4 cup feta cheese
- ✓ Black pepper to taste

Directions:

- ❖ Combine white beans, olives, lemon juice, arugula, onions, tuna, olive oil, and tomatoes in a mixing bowl.
- ❖ Sprinkle pepper and salt and feta cheese and serve.

Nutrition: Calories: 436 kcal Fat: 22 g Protein: 30 g Carbs: 39 g Fiber: 12 g

312) OUTRAGEOUS HERBACEOUS CHICKPEA SALAD IN ITALIAN STYLE

Preparation Time: 20 minutes	Cooking Time: 20 minutes	Servings: 4

Ingredients:

- ✓ 1/2 cup chopped celery with leaves
- ✓ 30 oz chickpeas
- ✓ 1.5 cups chopped parsley
- ✓ 1/2 cup chopped onion
- ✓ 3 tbsp olive oil
- ✓ 3 tbsp lemon juice
- ✓ Two minced cloves garlic
- ✓ 1/2 tsp kosher salt
- ✓ One chopped red bell pepper
- ✓ 1/2 tsp black pepper

Directions:

- ❖ Combine bell pepper, onion, chickpeas, celery, and parsley in a mixing bowl.
- ❖ In another bowl. Mix olive oil, garlic, salt, lemon juice, and pepper.
- ❖ Pour olive oil mixture over chickpeas mixture and mix well and serve.

Nutrition: Calories: 474 kcal Fat: 16 g Protein: 20 g Carbs: 65 g Fiber: 18 g

313) EASY AVOCADO CAPRESE SALAD

Preparation Time: 5 minutes	Cooking Time: 0 minute	Servings: 1

Ingredients:

- ✓ 1 cup sliced cherry tomatoes
- ✓ 1/4 cup basil leaves
- ✓ 1/2 cup mozzarella cheese balls
- ✓ ½ avocado
- ✓ 2 tsp extra virgin olive oil
- ✓ Salt to taste
- ✓ 2 tsp balsamic vinegar
- ✓ Black pepper to taste

Directions:

- ❖ In a bowl, combine cheese, tomatoes, avocado, olive oil, salt, basil, vinegar, and black pepper.
- ❖ Mix well and serve.

Nutrition: Calories: 456 kcal Fat: 37 g Protein: 17 g Carbs: 20 g Fiber: 9 g

314) TOMATO AND HEARTS OF PALM SALAD

Preparation Time: 15 minutes	Cooking Time: 0 minute	Servings: 4

Ingredients:

- ✓ 14 oz sliced hearts of palm, diced avocados tbsp lime juice cup sliced grape tomatoes
- ✓ 1/4 cup sliced green onion
- ✓ 1/2 cup chopped cilantro
- ✓ Salt to taste

Directions:

- ❖ In a bowl, combine drained and sliced palm hearts, lime juice, tomatoes, avocados, and onions.
- ❖ Mix salt to adjust the taste.
- ❖ Sprinkle cilantro to enhance the taste and serve.

Nutrition: Calories: 199 kcal Fat: 15 g Protein: 5 g Carbs: 15 g Fiber: 10 g

315) GREEK QUINOA TABBOULEH WITH CHICKPEAS

Preparation Time: 20 minutes	Cooking Time: 15 minutes	Servings: 8

✓ 1 cup quinoa ✓ 2 cups of water ✓ 1.5 cups chickpeas cooked cups sliced cherry tomatoescups slicing cucumber ✓ 3/4 cups chopped parsley	✓ 2/3 cups chopped onions Tbsp chopped mint ✓ Ground Pepper to taste ✓ Dressing ✓ 1/3 cups olive oil lemon zest tbsp lemon juice ✓ 1.5 tsp minced garlic ✓ ¾ tsp salt	❖ In a bowl, mix lemon juice, salt, oil, lemon zest, and garlic. The dressing is ready. ❖ In a deep pot, add two cups of water, a pinch of salt, and quinoa. Let it boil. ❖ When the water starts boiling, lower the flame to low and cover. Let it simmer for about 15 minutes. ❖ Strain quinoa and set aside to cool down. ❖ In a bowl, combine onions, cucumbers, mint, tomatoes, cooked quinoa, parsley, black pepper, and chickpeas. ❖ Add dressing in quinoa mixture and mix well. ❖ Adjust flavor using black pepper and salt and serve.

316) SPECIAL GREEK-STYLE AVOCADO SALAD

Preparation Time: 20 minutes	Cooking Time: 0 minute	Servings: 8

✓ Two sliced English cucumbers ✓ 1.5 lb chopped tomatoes ✓ 1/4 sliced red onion 1/2 cups sliced Kalamata olives ✓ 1/4 cup chopped parsleysliced avocados ✓ 1 cup feta cheese	✓ 1/2 cup extra virgin olive oil ✓ 1/2 cup red wine vinegar minced garlic cloves ✓ 1 tbsp oregano ✓ 2 tsp sugar ✓ 1 tsp kosher salt ✓ 1 tsp ground black pepper	❖ Mix tomatoes, parsley, onions, cucumbers, avocado, and olives. Set aside. ❖ Whisk vinegar, sugar, olive oil, salt, oregano, garlic, and pepper in a jar. Close the lid and shake to get the emulsified mixture. You can add salt, black pepper, and sugar to adjust the taste according to you. The dressing is ready. ❖ Transfer the dressing to the salad bowl and toss well. ❖ Garnish with feta cheese and serve.

317) EASY WINTER COUSCOUS SALAD

Preparation Time: 10 minutes	Cooking Time: 25 minutes	Servings: 8

✓ Salad ✓ 1.5 cups dry pearl couscous ✓ 2 lb cubed butternut squash ✓ 1/2 cup dried cranberries ✓ 1/2 chopped red onion ✓ sliced fennel bulb ✓ tbsp olive oil bunch sliced kale ✓ 1/2 cup chopped pecans	✓ Dressing ✓ 2 tbsp apple cider vinegar ✓ 1/3 cup olive oil ✓ 2 tbsp honey tbsp Dijon mustard ✓ 1 tbsp lemon juice ✓ Kosher salt to taste tbsp orange juice ✓ Black pepper to taste	❖ Put fennel, onions, and butternut squash over a baking tray lined with a parchment sheet. ❖ Sprinkle salt, olive oil, and black pepper over butternut squash. ❖ Bake in a preheated oven at 400 degrees for 30 minutes. ❖ Cook couscous by following the instructions given on the package. ❖ Mix mustard, olive oil, juice, vinegar, honey, salt, and black pepper in a jar and shake until the mixture emulsifies. The dressing is ready. ❖ In a bowl, combine baked veggies, kale, pecans, couscous, and cranberries. Pour dressing over the mixture and toss well. ❖ Serve and enjoy it.

318)   SLOW-COOKED ITALIAN CHICKEN CACCIATORE

Preparation Time: 15 minutes	Cooking Time: 240 minutes	Servings: 5

Ingredients	Ingredients	Directions
✓ Three chopped garlic cloves ✓ 1.5 tbsp olive oil ✓ 1.25 tbsp balsamic vinegar ✓ 1 tsp kosher salt ✓ 1/2 tsp black pepper ✓ 2 tsp Italian seasoning	✓ 28 oz crushed tomatoes ✓ 2 lb boneless chicken breastschopped yellow onion ✓ One chopped green bell pepper ✓ 8 oz sliced cremini mushrooms	❖ Rub the chicken with salt and black pepper and cook in heated oil in a skillet over a high flame for five minutes from both sides. ❖ Shift the chicken to the slow cooker. ❖ Sauté onions in heated oil for three minutes in a skillet over medium flame. ❖ Stir in vinegar and garlic and cook for one more minute. ❖ Shift the garlic mixture to the slow cooker. ❖ Add mushrooms, tomatoes, Italian seasoning, and bell pepper and mix. ❖ Cover the cooker and cook on low flame for four hours. ❖ After chicken is done, sprinkle salt, vinegar, and pepper and serve with rice or whatever you like.

Nutrition: Calories: 228 kcal Fat: 8 g Protein: 32 g Carbs: 10 g Fiber: 3 g

319)   GREEK STYLE BAKED COD WITH LEMON AND GARLIC

Preparation Time: 10 minutes	Cooking Time: 12 minutes	Servings: 4

Ingredients	Ingredients	Directions
✓ Five minced garlic cloves 1.5 lb Cod fillet ✓ ¼ cup chopped parsley ✓ Lemon Juice Mixture ✓ 5 tbsp Olive oil ✓ 5 tbsp lemon juice ✓ 2 tbsp butter	✓ Coating ✓ 1/3 cup all-purpose flour ✓ ¾ tsp salt ✓ ¾ tsp paprika 1 tsp coriander ✓ ¾ tsp cumin ✓ ½ tsp black pepper	❖ In a medium-sized bowl, combine olive oil, butter, and lemon juice and keep it aside. ❖ Whisk flour, salt, spices, and pepper in a bowl and keep it aside. ❖ Coat fish with lemon mixture followed by coating with flour mixture. ❖ Sauté coated fish in heated olive oil in a skillet over medium flame for two minutes from each side. ❖ Mix garlic into lemon juice and pour over sautéed fish. ❖ Bake in a preheated oven at 400 degrees for almost 10 minutes. ❖ Drizzle parsley and serve with your favorite salad or rice.

Nutrition: Calories: 312 kcal Fat: 18.4 g Protein: 23.1 g Carbs: 16.1 g Fiber: 14 g

320)   EASY BAKED HALIBUT AND VEGETABLES IN ONE PAN

Preparation Time: 10 minutes	Cooking Time: 15 minutes	Servings: 6

Ingredients	Ingredients	Directions
✓ For the Sauce: ✓ Zest of two lemons tsp dried oregano ✓ ½ tsp black pepper ✓ 1 cup Olive oil ✓ 4 tbsp lemon juice ✓ 1 tsp seasoned salt tbsp minced garlic tsp dill ✓ ¾ tsp coriander	✓ For the Fish ✓ sliced yellow onion ✓ 1 lb green beans lb sliced halibut fillet ✓ 1 lb cherry tomatoes	❖ Whisk olive oil, onions, oregano, salt, dill, pepper, tomatoes, lemon zest, green beans, juice, coriander, and garlic in a bowl. ❖ Spread vegetable mixture over one side of the baking tray. ❖ Coat halibut fillets with the sauce and place them on a baking tray. ❖ Pour the leftover sauce over the vegetable mixture and fillets. ❖ Bake in a preheated oven at 425 degrees for 15 minutes.

Nutrition: Calories: 390 kcal Fat: 31.3 g Protein: 17.5 g Carbs: 8.8 g Fiber: 4.1 g

321) AFRICAN MOROCCAN FISH

Preparation Time: 10 minutes	Cooking Time: 30 minutes	Servings: 6

✓ Olive oil as required ✓ 2 tbsp tomato paste ✓ Eight minced garlic cloves ✓ Two diced tomatoes ✓ ½ tsp cumin ✓ 15 oz chickpeas sliced red pepper cup water	✓ Kosher salt to taste ✓ Handful of cilantros ✓ Black pepper to taste ✓ 1.5 lb cod fillet pieces ✓ 1.5 tsp allspice mixture ✓ ¾ tsp paprika ✓ 1 tbsp lemon juice ✓ ½ sliced lemon	❖ Sauté garlic in heated oil for one minute. ❖ Stir in bell pepper and diced tomatoes and tomato paste and cook for five minutes over medium flame with constant stirring. ❖ Mix garlic, salt, chickpeas, cilantro, pepper, water, and half tsp of allspice mixture. Let it boil and reduce the flame and simmer for 20 minutes. ❖ Whisk leftover allspice mixture, paprika, salt, cumin, and pepper in a bowl. ❖ Rub fish with spice mixture and oil. ❖ Place fish and fish mixture in a pan, followed by a cooked chickpea mixture, lemon slices, and juice. ❖ Let it cook for 15 minutes over low flame. ❖ Sprinkle cilantro and serve. ❖ Sprinkle spice mixture over the fish

322) ITALIAN STYLE BAKED CHICKEN

Preparation Time: 10 minutes	Cooking Time: 18 minutes	Servings: 6

✓ 2 lb boneless chicken breast ✓ Pepper to taste tsp thyme ✓ One sliced red onion tsp dry oregano ✓ 1 tsp sweet paprika tbsp olive oil minced garlic cloves	✓ 1 tbsp of lemon juice halved Campari tomatoes ✓ Salt to taste ✓ Handful chopped parsley for garnishing ✓ Basil leaves as required for garnishing	❖ Flatten the chicken pieces suing meat mallet in a zip lock bag. ❖ Rub chicken pieces with black pepper and salt and add them to the bowl. Add lemon juice, garlic, oil, and spices and mix well to fully coat the chicken. ❖ Place onions in an oiled baking tray followed by chicken and tomatoes. ❖ Bake in a preheated oven at 425 degrees for 10 minutes while covering the tray with foil. ❖ After ten minutes, uncover and bake again for eight more minutes. ❖ Serve after sprinkle parsley over the baked chicken.

323) SPECIAL LEMON GARLIC SALMON

Preparation Time: 10 minutes	Cooking Time: 18 minutes	Servings: 6

✓ Salmon ✓ 2 lb salmon fillet ✓ 2 tbsp parsley for garnishing ✓ Olive oil ✓ Kosher salt ✓ ½ sliced lemon	✓ Lemon-Garlic Sauce ✓ Zest of one lemon ✓ 3 tbsp olive oil ✓ 3 tbsp of lemon juice ✓ Five chopped garlic cloves tsp sweet paprika tsp dry oregano ✓ ½ tsp black pepper	❖ In a bowl, whisk olive oil, pepper, garlic, lemon zest and juice, oregano, and paprika in a mixing bowl and set aside. The lemon garlic sauce is ready. ❖ Brush baking tray with oil lined with foil paper. ❖ Place seasoned (with salt) salmon on a baking tray and pour the sauce over the salmon. ❖ Bake in a preheated oven at 375 degrees for 20 minutes. ❖ Broil baked salmon for three minutes and serve after garnishing.

324) PAN-FRIED CHICKEN AND VEGETABLES

Preparation Time: 15 minutes	**Cooking Time:** 45 minutes	**Servings:** 6

✓ 2 lb red potatoes ✓ 2 tbsp olive oil ✓ One chopped onion ✓ Three minced garlic cloves ✓ 1 tsp powdered rosemary	✓ .25 tsp salt ✓ 3/4 tsp pepper ✓ Six chicken thighs ✓ 1/2 tsp paprika ✓ 6 cups baby spinach	❖ Mix onion, rosemary, potatoes, oil, salt, garlic, and pepper in a bowl. Shift the potato mixture into a baking tray sprayed with oil. ❖ Combine salt, pepper, paprika, and rosemary in another bowl and sprinkle over chicken. Place chicken pieces over potato mixture and bake in a preheated oven at 425 degrees for 35 minutes. ❖ Take chicken out of oven and place in serving dish. Put spinach over veggies and bake for another ten minutes. Transfer cooked veggies over chicken and serve.

325) SICILIAN FISH STEW

Preparation Time: 10 minutes	**Cooking Time:** 35 minutes	**Servings:** 6

✓ Olive oil ✓ Two chopped celery ribs chopped yellow onion ✓ Salt to taste ✓ Four minced garlic cloves tbsp toasted pine nuts ✓ Black pepper to taste ✓ ½ tsp dried thyme ✓ ¾ cup dry white wine	✓ One pinch of red pepper flakes ✓ 28 oz plum tomatoes ✓ Tomato juice ✓ ¼ cup golden raisins cups vegetable broth ✓ 2 tbsp capers ✓ ½ cup chopped parsley leaves ✓ 2 lb sliced skinless bass fillet ✓ Italian bread for serving	❖ Sauté onions and celery, black pepper, and salt in a Dutch oven over medium flame with constant stirring for four minutes. ❖ Add flakes, thyme, and garlic, and cook for one minute. ❖ Mix tomato juice and white wine and let it simmer. ❖ When the liquid is concentrated to half, add capers, tomatoes, raisins, and stock. ❖ Cook for 20 more minutes. ❖ Rub fish with pepper and salt and add in cooking solution and mix well. Let it simmer for five minutes. ❖ Remove from the flame and let it cool for five minutes while the oven is covered. ❖ Sprinkle parsley and pine nuts and serve.

326) SPECIAL GREEK CHICKEN SOUVLAKI

Preparation Time: 45 minutes	**Cooking Time:** 40 minutes	**Servings:** 4

✓ Margination ✓ 12 boneless chicken thighs ✓ 4 tbsp olive oil tsp dried mint tsp dried oregano ✓ 1 tsp ground cumin ✓ 1 tsp sweet paprika crushed garlic cloves ✓ 1 tsp coriander ✓ ½ tsp ground cinnamon ✓ 1 tbsp lemon juice ✓ Zest of one lemon ✓ Wedges cut slices of one lemon slices	✓ Pitta wraps ✓ 250 g white bread flour tsp caster sugar ✓ 7 g dried yeast tsp olive oil ✓ Tzatziki sauce ✓ crushed garlic clove ✓ ½ chopped cucumber small bunch of chopped mint leaves ✓ 200 g Greek yogurt ✓ 1 tbsp lemon juice ✓ To serve ✓ Four chopped tomatoes One lettuce ✓ One sliced red onion	❖ In a large mixing bowl, add chicken and black pepper, salt, and all the ingredients mentioned in the marination list. Toss to coat well. Leave it overnight for better results in the refrigerator. ❖ Whisk flour, sugar, salt, and yeast in a bowl. Pour 2 tsp oil and warm water about 150 ml and mix to form a dough. Knead the dough for ten minutes. ❖ Cover the bowl and set aside for 60 minutes. ❖ Make four portions of the raised dough, roll them into circles, and set aside 20 more minutes. The dough for pita bread is ready. ❖ In a bowl, mix all the ingredients of the Tzatziki sauce and set aside. The Tzatziki sauce is ready. ❖ Thread chicken pieces on skewers separately, place the skewers over the top of roasting tin, place overheated grill, and cook the chicken for 20 minutes while brushing with oil. When chicken is done, set aside. ❖ Brush the flattened pita bread with oil and place in a heated pan. Cook for three minutes, and when it turned golden from the underside, then flip and cook the other side for three more minutes. When the bread is fully cooked, cover it and keep it warm until further use. ❖ Make kebabs out of grilled chicken and place in pita bread followed by tomato, onion, lettuce, lemon slices, and drizzle Tzatziki sauce and serve.

Nutrition: Calories: 707 kcal Fat: 34 g Protein: 46 g Carbs: 52 g Fiber: 4 g

327)   EASY GRILLED SWORDFISH

Preparation Time: 15 minutes	Cooking Time: 8 minutes	Servings: 4

Ingredients:

- ✓ Ten garlic cloves
- ✓ 2 tbsp lemon juice
- ✓ 1/3 cup olive oil 2 tsp coriander
- ✓ 1 tsp Spanish paprika
- ✓ ¾ tsp cumin
- ✓ ¾ tsp salt
- ✓ Four swordfish steaks
- ✓ ½ tsp black pepper
- ✓ Crushed red pepper to taste

Directions:

- ❖ Blend olive oil, pepper, garlic, salt, and lemon juice in a blender to obtain a smooth mixture.
- ❖ Coat swordfish with the garlic blended mixture and keep it aside for 15 minutes.
- ❖ Heat grill on high flame. Place fish and cook for five minutes from each side.
- ❖ Sprinkle lemon juice and flakes and serve.

328)   GREEK STYLE PRAWNS WITH TOMATOES AND FETA CHEESE

Preparation Time: 10 minutes	Cooking Time: 40 minutes	Servings: 4

Ingredients:

- ✓ 4 tbsp olive oil
- ✓ 3/4 cup chopped shallots
- ✓ Four chopped garlic cloves
- ✓ 28 oz diced tomatoes 1 tsp salt
- ✓ 1/4 tsp pepper 2 tsp cumin
- ✓ 1/2 tsp crushed pepper flakes
- ✓ 1 tbsp honey
- ✓ 1.5 lb shrimp
- ✓ 6 oz feta cheese
- ✓ 3/4 tsp dried oregano 2 tbsp chopped mint

Directions:

- ❖ Cook garlic and shallots in heated oil in a skillet over low flame for eight minutes.
- ❖ Stir in salt, cumin, honey, tomatoes, tomato juices, flakes, and pepper.
- ❖ Let the sauce boil and cook for 20 minutes with occasional stirring.
- ❖ Remove from flame and add shrimps in the sauce. Sprinkle feta cheese and oregano.
- ❖ Bake in a preheated oven at 400 degrees for 15 minutes.
- ❖ Shift the shrimp pan to broil and broil for two minutes.
- ❖ Garnish with mint and serve.

329)   SIMPLE SALMON KABOBS

Preparation Time: 10 minutes	Cooking Time: 8 minutes	Servings: 6

Ingredients:

- ✓ 1.5 lb sliced Salmon fillet
- ✓ One sliced red onion
- ✓ One sliced zucchini
- ✓ Kosher salt to taste
- ✓ Black pepper to taste
- ✓ Marinade
- ✓ 1/3 cup Olive Oil
- ✓ Zest of one lemon 2 tbsp lemon juice minced garlic cloves
- ✓ 1 tsp chili pepper 2 tsp dry oregano
- ✓ 2 tsp chopped thyme leaves
- ✓ 1 tsp cumin
- ✓ ½ tsp coriander

Directions:

- ❖ Mix all the ingredients of margination in a bowl.
- ❖ In another bowl, add pepper, onions, salt, salmon, and zucchini and mix well.
- ❖ Add marinade and mix well. Set aside for 20 minutes.
- ❖ Thread onions, salmon, and zucchini in skewers.
- ❖ Place skewers overheated grill, cover them, and grill for eight minutes.
- ❖ When salmons are ready, serve and enjoy it.

Nutrition: Calories: 267 kcal Fat: 11 g Protein: 35 g Carbs: 7 g Fiber: 3 g

330) ORIGINAL SAUTEED SHRIMP AND ZUCCHINI

Preparation Time: 8 minutes	Cooking Time: 7 minutes	Servings: 3

Ingredients:

- lb shrimp
- 1 tsp salt Two zucchinis 2 tbsp chopped garlic
- 1 tbsp butter
- ✓ Black pepper to taste 1.5 tbsp lemon juice
- ✓ 2 tbsp chopped parsley
- ✓ Olive oil as required

❖ Add salt, shrimps, and pepper in a bowl. Mix them well.
❖ Cook shrimps in heated oil over medium flame for two minutes from each side. Shift cooked shrimps in a plate.
❖ Cook zucchini in heated oil in the same pan for two minutes, then sprinkle pepper and salt.
❖ Transfer shrimps to the pan and mix. Add garlic and sauté for two minutes.
❖ Add butter and cook to melt it.
❖ When shrimps, garlic, and zucchini are cooked, add lemon juice and mix well.
❖ Drizzle parsley and serve.

331) GREEK-STYLE CHICKEN AND POTATOES

Preparation Time: 10 minutes	Cooking Time: 50 minutes	Servings: 4

- ✓ 4 lb chicken thighs 2 tbsp oregano
- ✓ 1 tbsp salt
- ✓ 1 tsp black pepper
- ✓ 2/3 cup chicken stock
- ✓ One pinch of cayenne pepper
- ✓ 1 tsp rosemary
- ✓ ½ cup lemon juice
- ✓ Six minced garlic cloves
- ✓ ½ cup olive oil
- ✓ Three sliced russet potatoes
- ✓ 1 tbsp chopped oregano

❖ Add lemon juice, oregano, oil, cayenne pepper, salt, garlic, rosemary, black pepper potatoes, and chicken in a bowl. Mix them to coat everything well.
❖ Place chicken in a roasting tray.
❖ Spread potato pieces, 2/3 cup of stock, and marinade over chicken pieces.
❖ Bake in a preheated oven at 425 degrees for 20 minutes.
❖ Change the sides of the chicken and bake for 20 more minutes.
❖ Bake until chicken is done and shift chicken in serving dish.
❖ Mix potatoes with remaining juice and broil for three minutes.
❖ Shift the potatoes in the serving dish beside the chicken.
❖ Concentrate chicken stock left in a roasting tray on the stove over medium flame.

332) EASY ITALIAN BAKED FISH

Preparation Time: 5 minutes	Cooking Time: 30 minutes	Servings: 6

- ✓ 1/3 cup olive oil
- ✓ Two diced tomatoes 1.5 chopped red onion
- ✓ Ten chopped garlic cloves
- ✓ 1 tsp Spanish paprika 2 tsp coriander
- ✓ 1 tsp cumin
- ✓ 1.5 tbsp capers
- ✓ ½ tsp cayenne pepper
- ✓ Salt to taste
- ✓ 1/3 cup raisins
- ✓ 1 tbsp of lemon juice
- ✓ Black pepper to taste
- ✓ Parsley for garnishing
- ✓ Zest of one lemon
- ✓ 1.5 lb white fish fillet
- ✓ Mint for garnishing

❖ Cook onions in heated olive oil in a saucepan for three minutes.
❖ Stir in tomatoes, salt, capers, garlic, raisins, and spices and let them boil.
❖ Reduce the flame to low and simmer for 15 minutes.
❖ Rub fish with pepper and salt and set aside.
❖ Transfer half of the cooked tomato mixture to the baking pan, followed by fish, lemon juice, zest, and leftover tomato mixture.
❖ Bake in a preheated oven at 400 degrees for 18 minutes.
❖ Sprinkle mint and parsley and serve.

Nutrition: Calories: 308 kcal Fat: 17.4 g Protein: 27 g Carbs: 13.3 g Fiber: 2 g

333) SPECIAL GREEK TZATZIKI SAUCE AND DIP

Preparation Time: 10 minutes	Cooking Time: 0 minute	Servings: 4

Ingredients:

- ✓ ½ halved cucumber
- ✓ 3/4 cup Yogurt
- ✓ Two minced garlic cloves2 tbsp red wine vinegar
- ✓ 1 tbsp minced dill
- ✓ One pinch of kosher salt
- ✓ One pinch of black pepper

Directions:

- ❖ Place dried shredded cucumber in a bowl.
- ❖ Mix garlic, vinegar, salt, yogurt, dill, and pepper in cucumber and mix well.
- ❖ Cover the bowl and place it in the refrigerator. The Tzatziki sauce is ready.
- ❖ Can store up to three days.

Nutrition: Calories: 30 kcal Fat: 1 g Protein: 4 g Carbs: 3 g Fiber: 1 g

334) ITALIAN PESTO AND GARLIC SHRIMP BRUSCHETTA

Preparation Time: 10 minutes	Cooking Time: 15 minutes	Servings: 12

Ingredients:

- ✓ 8 oz shrimp
- ✓ Black pepper to taste
- ✓ 2 tbsp butter
- ✓ 4 tbsp olive oil
- ✓ 20 basil leaves One bread
- ✓ Four minced garlic cloves3 oz pesto
- ✓ 2 oz capers3 oz sun-dried tomatoes
- ✓ 1 oz feta cheese
- ✓ kosher salt to taste
- ✓ Glaze Balsamic for garnishing

Directions:

- ❖ Sprinkle salt and pepper over shrimps in a bowl. Set aside for ten minutes.
- ❖ Add olive oil and butter of about 2 tbsp each in the pan and cook for 2 minutes over medium flame.
- ❖ Stir in garlic and sauté for one more minute.
- ❖ Mix shrimps and cook for four minutes.
- ❖ Remove from flame and let it set.
- ❖ Slice the bread and place in a baking tray and drizzle oil and toast in the oven for five minutes.
- ❖ Spread pesto sauce over each bread slice followed by sun-dried tomatoes, shrimp, caper, cheese, basil, and balsamic glaze and serve.

Nutrition: Calories: 168 kcal Fat: 7 g Protein: 5 g Carbs: 19 g Fiber: 1 g

335) EASY PAN-SEARED CITRUS SHRIMP

Preparation Time: 5 minutes	Cooking Time: 10 minutes	Servings: 6

Ingredients:

- ✓ 1 tbsp olive oil
- ✓ 6 tbsp cup lemon juice
- ✓ 1 cup of orange juice
- ✓ One sliced orange
- ✓ Five minced garlic cloves
- ✓ 1 tbsp chopped parsley
- ✓ 1 tbsp chopped red onion
- ✓ One pinch of red pepper flakes
- ✓ Kosher salt to taste
- ✓ Black pepper to taste 3 lb shrimp
- ✓ One wedge cut lemon

Directions:

- ❖ Mix parsley, pepper flakes, orange juice, oil, garlic, lemon juice, and onions in a bowl.
- ❖ Transfer the onion mixture to skillet and cook over medium flame for eight minutes.
- ❖ Add salt, pepper, and shrimps in a skillet and cook for five minutes or until shrimps are done.
- ❖ Garnish with parsley and lemon slices and serve.

Nutrition: Calories: 291 kcal Fat: 6 g Protein: 47 g Carbs: 11 g Fiber: 1 g

336)   SIMPLE CUCUMBER AND TOMATO SALAD

Preparation Time: 10 minutes	Cooking Time: 0 minute	Servings: 4

Ingredients:

- ✓ One sliced English cucumber
- ✓ ½ sliced red onion
- ✓ Three diced tomatoes
- ✓ 2 tbsp olive oil
- ✓ Salt to taste
- ✓ 1 tbsp red wine vinegar
- ✓ Black pepper to taste

Directions:

- ❖ In a large mixing bowl, mix all the ingredients and place in the refrigerator for 20 minutes.
- ❖ Serve and enjoy it.

Nutrition: Calories: 104 kcal Fat: 8 g Protein: 2 g Carbs: 7 g Fiber: 2 g

337)   EASY CITRUS AVOCADO DIP

Preparation Time: 15 minutes	Cooking Time: 0 minute	Servings: 8

Ingredients:

- ✓ Two diced oranges
- ✓ ½ cup chopped onions
- ✓ ½ cup chopped mint
- ✓ ½ cup chopped cilantro
- ✓ Olive oil as required
- ✓ Two sliced avocados
- ✓ ½ cup chopped walnuts
- ✓ Black pepper to taste
- ✓ Cayenne as required
- ✓ Salt to taste
- ✓ 1 tbsp of lime juice
- ✓ ¾ tsp sumac
- ✓ 1.75 oz shredded feta cheese

Directions:

- ❖ In a bowl, combine all the ingredients and mix well.
- ❖ Serve and enjoy it.

Nutrition: Calories: 147 kcal Fat: 10.3 g Protein: 2.8 g Carbs: 14.6 g Fiber: 2.1 g

338)   ROASTED TOMATOES WITH THYME AND FETA CHEESE

Preparation Time: 5 minutes	Cooking Time: 20 minutes	Servings: 4

Ingredients:

- ✓ ½ tsp dried thyme
- ✓ 16 oz cherry tomatoes
- ✓ Black pepper to taste
- ✓ 3 tbsp olive oil
- ✓ Salt to taste
- ✓ 6 tbsp feta cheese

Directions:

- ❖ In a baking tray, put tomatoes.
- ❖ Pour olive oil and drizzle pepper, thyme leaves, and salt over tomatoes and mix well.
- ❖ Bake in a preheated oven at 450 degrees for 15 minutes.
- ❖ Drizzle cheese and broil for five minutes and serve when the cheese melts.

Nutrition: Calories: 195 kcal Fat: 7.3 g Protein: 2 g Carbs: 3.1 g Fiber: 1.1 g

339) ITALIAN BAKED ZUCCHINI WITH THYME AND PARMESAN

Preparation Time: 10 minutes	Cooking Time: 20 minutes	Servings: 4

Ingredients:

- ✓ Four sliced zucchinis
- ✓ 1/2 tsp dried thyme
- ✓ 1/2 cup shredded Parmesan cheese
- ✓ 1/2 tsp dried oregano
- ✓ 2 tbsp olive oil
- ✓ 1/4 tsp garlic powder
- ✓ Kosher salt to taste
- ✓ 1/2 tsp dried basil
- ✓ Black pepper to taste
- ✓ 2 tbsp chopped parsley

Directions:

- ❖ Mix all the ingredients in a large bowl except zucchini.
- ❖ Make a layer of zucchini over a baking sheet sprayed with oil.
- ❖ Transfer the cheese mixture over zucchini and pour olive oil over them.
- ❖ Bake in a preheated oven at 350 degrees for 15 minutes, followed by broiling for three minutes.
- ❖ Serve and enjoy it.

340) ITALIAN BABA GANOUSH

Preparation Time: 10 minutes	Cooking Time: 40 minutes	Servings: 4

Ingredients:

- ✓ One eggplant
- ✓ 1 tbsp Greek yogurt
- ✓ olive oil
- ✓ 1.5 tbsp tahini paste
- ✓ 1 tbsp lime juice
- ✓ One garlic clove
- ✓ Salt to taste
- ✓ 1 tsp cayenne pepper
- ✓ Pepper to taste
- ✓ ½ tsp sumac for garnishing
- ✓ Parsley leaves for garnishing
- ✓ Toasted pine nuts for garnishing

Directions:

- ❖ Make slits in eggplant's skin.
- ❖ Place eggplant skin side upwards in a baking tray.
- ❖ Spray olive oil over eggplant.
- ❖ Bake in a preheated oven at 425 degrees for 40 minutes.
- ❖ Scoop the inner flesh of eggplant out and shift in a food processor. Add garlic, cayenne, yogurt, lime juice, salt, tahini, sumac, pepper, and blend. The baba ganoush is ready.
- ❖ You can refrigerator for better results for 60 minutes and sprinkle oil, sumac, parsley, and nuts and serve.

341) SICILIAN SALMON FISH STICKS

Preparation Time: 10 minutes	Cooking Time: 18 minutes	Servings: 4

Ingredients:

- ✓ Fish Sticks
- ✓ 2 lb salmon fillet
- ✓ 1/4 tsp salt
- ✓ 1/4 tsp black pepper
- ✓ First coating
- ✓ 1/2 tsp garlic powder
- ✓ 1/2 tsp dried thyme
- ✓ 1 cup almond meal
- ✓ 1/2 tsp sea salt
- ✓ 1/4 tsp black pepper
- ✓ Second coating
- ✓ 1/2 tsp salt
- ✓ 2/3 cup chickpea flour
- ✓ Third coating
- ✓ Two eggs
- ✓ Dipping Sauce
- ✓ 1/4 tsp salt
- ✓ 1/4 cup Greek yogurt
- ✓ 1 tsp lemon juice
- ✓ 1 tbsp Dijon mustard
- ✓ 1/2 tsp dill
- ✓ 1/8 tsp garlic powder

Directions:

- ❖ Whisk all the ingredients for the dipping sauce list in a bowl and set aside. The dipping sauce is ready.
- ❖ Mix garlic, thyme, and almond meal in a bowl. The first coating is ready.
- ❖ Add chickpea flour in another bowl. The second coating is ready.
- ❖ Beat the eggs in another bowl. Set aside.
- ❖ Sprinkle pepper and salt over sliced fish with removed skin.
- ❖ First, coat the fish with chickpea flour, followed by coating with egg and almond meal coating.
- ❖ Aline coated fish pieces in a baking sheet covered with parchment paper.
- ❖ Bake in a preheated oven at 400 degrees for 18 minutes.
- ❖ Serve baked fish with dipping sauce and serve.

Nutrition: Calories: 92 kcal Fat: 5.7 g Protein: 14.4 g Carbs: 4.5 g Fiber: 1.3 g

342) AFRICAN BAKED FALAFEL

Preparation Time: 10 minutes	Cooking Time: 24 minutes	Servings: 15 patties

Ingredients:

- ✓ 15 oz chickpeas
- ✓ Three cloves garlic
- ✓ 1/4 cup chopped onion
- ✓ 1/2 cup parsley
- ✓ 2 tsp lemon juice
- ✓ 1/2 tsp baking soda
- ✓ 1 tbsp olive oil
- ✓ 1 tsp ground cumin
- ✓ 3/4 tsp salt
- ✓ 1 tsp coriander
- ✓ One pinch of cayenne
- ✓ 3 tbsp oat flour

Directions:

- ❖ Blend all the ingredients except oat flour and baking soda in a food processor to get roughly a blended mixture.
- ❖ Transfer the mixture to a bowl and add oat flour and baking soda. Using hands, mix the dough well.
- ❖ Make patties out of the falafel mixture and set aside for 15 minutes.
- ❖ Bake the falafel patties in a preheated oven at 375 degrees for 12 minutes and serve.

Nutrition: Calories: 143 kcal Fat: 5 g Protein: 6 g Carbs: 24 g Fiber: 6 g

343) GREEK CHIA YOGURT PUDDING

Preparation Time: 10 minutes	Cooking Time: 0 minute	Servings: 4

Ingredients:

- ✓ 3/4 cup milk
- ✓ 11 oz f Vanilla Yogurt
- ✓ 2 tbsp pure maple syrup
- ✓ 1 tsp vanilla extract
- ✓ 1/8 tsp salt
- ✓ 1/4 cup chia seeds
- ✓ Sliced almonds for garnishing

Directions:

- ❖ Whisk all the ingredients in a large bowl. Set aside for 24 hours in the refrigerator.
- ❖ Mix the mixture gently after 24 hours and serve after garnishing.

Nutrition: Calories: 179 kcal Fat: 5.6 g Protein: 10.1 g Carbs: 22.3 g Fiber: 6 g

344) EASY ITALIAN-STYLE FARFALLE

Preparation Time: 10 minutes	Cooking Time: 15 minutes	Servings: 7

Ingredients:

- ✓ 12 oz farfalle pasta
- ✓ ½ cup olive oil
- ✓ ¼ cup chopped basil leaves
- ✓ 1 lb crumbled chorizo sausage
- ✓ ½ cup pine nuts
- ✓ ½ cup shredded parmesan cheese
- ✓ Two chopped garlic cloves
- ✓ 1 cup diced tomato
- ✓ ¼ cup red wine vinegar

Directions:

- ❖ In a saucepan, boil water with added salt.
- ❖ Add pasta and cook until pasta is done.
- ❖ In a pan, cook chorizo over medium flame. Stir in nuts and cook for five minutes.
- ❖ Mix garlic and cook for a minute before removing the pan from the flame.
- ❖ Transfer cooked pasta, vinegar, cheese, cooked chorizo mixture, olive oil, tomatoes, and basil. Mix well to coat everything and serve.

Nutrition: Calories: 692 kcal Fat: 48 g Protein: 26.9 g Carbs: 39.7 g Fiber: 15 g

345)   SPECIAL POTATO WEDGES

Preparation Time: 5 minutes	Cooking Time: 30 minutes	Servings: 4

Ingredients:

- ✓ Two wedges cut potatoes
- ✓ ½ tsp salt
- ✓ ½ tsp paprika
- ✓ 1.5 tbsp olive oil
- ✓ ½ tsp chili powder
- ✓ 1/8 black pepper

Directions:

- ❖ Combine all the ingredients in a bowl.
- ❖ Transfer the mixture to an air fryer basket and cook in a preheated air fryer at 400 degrees for eight minutes from both sides.
- ❖ Serve and enjoy it.

346)   ORIGINAL GREEK-STYLE POTATOES

Preparation Time: 20 minutes	Cooking Time: 120 minutes	Servings: 4

Ingredients:

- ✓ 1/3 cup olive oil
- ✓ Two chopped garlic cloves
- ✓ 1.5 cups water
- ✓ Black pepper to taste
- ✓ ¼ cup lemon juice
- ✓ 1 tsp rosemary
- ✓ 1 tsp thyme
- ✓ Two chicken bouillon cubes
- ✓ Six chopped potatoes

Directions:

- ❖ Mix all the ingredients in a large bowl and pour over the potatoes placed in the baking tray.
- ❖ Bake in a preheated oven at 350 degrees for 90 minutes.
- ❖ Serve and enjoy it.

347)   ORGINIAL ITALIAN-STYLE CHICKEN WRAP

Preparation Time: 10 minutes	Cooking Time: 20 minutes	Servings: 4

Ingredients:

- ✓ 2 tbsp butter
- ✓ 1/2 cup mayonnaise
- ✓ 1/2 lb boneless chicken breasts
- ✓ 1/4 cup shredded Parmesan cheese
- ✓ 2 cups shredded romaine lettuce
- ✓ Four flour tortillas
- ✓ Two sliced Roma tomatoes
- ✓ 1/2 cup crushed croutons
- ✓ 16 basil leaves

Directions:

- ❖ Cook chicken over medium flame in melted butter for 20 minutes.
- ❖ Slice the chicken into strips.
- ❖ Whisk cheese and mayonnaise and pour over the tortilla.
- ❖ Place lettuce followed by chicken, basil, tomato, and croutons on tortilla and wrap.
- ❖ Serve and enjoy it.

348)   Lovely Avocado Caprese wrap

Preparation Time: 20 minutes	Cooking Time: 0 minute	Servings: 3

- ✓ Two tortillas
- ✓ Balsamic vinegar as needed
- ✓ One ball mozzarella cheese grated
- ✓ 1/2 cup arugula leaves
- ✓ One sliced tomato
- ✓ 2 tbsp basil leaves
- ✓ Kosher salt to taste
- ✓ One sliced avocado
- ✓ Olive oil as required
- ✓ Black pepper to taste

Directions:

- ❖ Place tomato slices and cheese, followed by avocado and basil. Over one side of the tortilla.
- ❖ Pour olive oil and vinegar. Drizzle pepper and salt.
- ❖ Wrap the tortilla and serve.

349) DELICIOUS CHICKEN SALAD WITH AVOCADO AND GREEK YOGURT

Preparation Time: 10 minutes	Cooking Time: 0 minute	Servings: 4

Ingredients:

- ✓ 1 cup plain yogurt
- ✓ 1 tbsp lemon juice
- ✓ One mashed avocado
- ✓ 1/3 cup dried cranberries
- ✓ Kosher salt to taste
- ✓ 2 cups shredded chicken
- ✓ Black pepper to taste
- ✓ 3/4 cup chopped celery
- ✓ 1/3 cup chopped pecans
- ✓ 1/2 cup chopped red grapes
- ✓ 1/3 cup chopped red onion
- ✓ 2 tbsp chopped tarragon

Directions:

- ❖ Whisk all the ingredients in a large mixing bowl.
- ❖ Serve as a salad and enjoy it.

350) EASY CHICKEN SHAWARMA PITAS

Preparation Time: 10 minutes	Cooking Time: 30 minutes	Servings: 6

- ✓ ¾ tbsp cumin
- ✓ ¾ tbsp coriander
- ✓ ¾ tbsp turmeric powder
- ✓ One sliced onion
- ✓ ¾ tbsp garlic powder
- ✓ ½ tsp cloves
- ✓ ¾ tbsp paprika
- ✓ 1 tbsp lemon juice
- ✓ ½ tsp cayenne pepper
- ✓ Eight boneless chicken
- ✓ Salt to taste
- ✓ 1/3 cup olive oil
- ✓ Pita bread
- ✓ Tahini sauce

Directions:

- ❖ In a bowl, add sliced chicken pieces, onions, cumin, garlic, cloves, olive oil, turmeric, paprika, lemon juice, salt, and coriander. Toss well to coat chicken evenly. Set aside for three hours in the refrigerator.
- ❖ Transfer the chicken pieces along with the marinade in a baking tray sprayed with oil.
- ❖ Bake in a preheated oven at 425 degrees for 30 minutes.
- ❖ Spread tahini sauce in pita bread and add baked chicken pieces. You can also add your favorite salad.
- ❖ Serve and enjoy it.

351) SIMPLE RED LENTIL SOUP

Preparation Time: 10 minutes	Cooking Time: 45 minutes	Servings: 4

- ✓ Four minced garlic cloves
- ✓ ¼ cup olive oil
- ✓ 1 tsp curry powder
- ✓ Two chopped carrots
- ✓ 2 tsp ground cumin
- ✓ One chopped onion
- ✓ ½ tsp dried thyme
- ✓ 1 cup brown lentils
- ✓ 28 oz diced tomatoes
- ✓ 4 cups vegetable broth
- ✓ 1 tsp salt
- ✓ 2 cups of water
- ✓ One pinch of red pepper flakes
- ✓ 1 cup chopped kale
- ✓ Black pepper to taste
- ✓ 1.5 tbsp lemon juice

Directions:

- ❖ Cook carrots and onions in ¼ cup of heated olive oil in a Dutch oven over medium flame for five minutes.
- ❖ Stir in thyme, cumin, garlic, and curry powder,
- ❖ Cook for half a minute.
- ❖ Add tomatoes and cook for another five minutes.
- ❖ Add pepper flakes, broth, salt, lentils, black pepper, and water in a Dutch oven.
- ❖ Let it boil. Cover the oven and lower the flame and let it simmer for 30 minutes.
- ❖ Blend a portion of soup of about two cups in a food processor and transfer it into the pot again.
- ❖ Mix chopped greens and cook for another five minutes.
- ❖ Remove from the flame and mix lemon juice and serve.

Nutrition: Calories: 366 kcal Fat: 15.5 g Protein: 14.5 g Carbs: 47.8 g Fiber: 10.8 g

352) EASY SALMON SOUP

Preparation Time: 10 minutes	Cooking Time: 12 minutes	Servings: 4

Ingredients:

- ✓ Olive oil
- ✓ ½ chopped green bell pepper
- ✓ Four chopped green onions
- ✓ Four minced garlic cloves
- ✓ 5 cups chicken broth
- ✓ 1 oz chopped dill
- ✓ 1 lb sliced gold potatoes
- ✓ 1 tsp dry oregano
- ✓ One sliced carrot
- ✓ ¾ tsp coriander
- ✓ Kosher salt to taste
- ✓ ½ tsp cumin
- ✓ Black pepper to taste
- ✓ Zest of one lemon
- ✓ 1 lb sliced salmon fillet
- ✓ 1 tbsp lemon juice

Directions:

- ❖ Cook onions, garlic, and bell pepper in heated olive oil in a pot over medium flame for four minutes.
- ❖ Stir in the dill and cook for half a minute.
- ❖ Pour broth into the pot. Add carrot, potatoes, salt, spices, and pepper.
- ❖ Let it boil. Reduce the flame and let it simmer for six minutes.
- ❖ Add salmon and cook for five more minutes.
- ❖ Add lemon juice and zest and cook for one minute.
- ❖ Serve the soup and enjoy it.

353) RICH FALAFEL SANDWICHES

Preparation Time: 20 minutes	Cooking Time: 10 minutes	Servings: 4 sandwiches

Ingredients:

- ✓ 4 Pita Breads
- ✓ 1 cup arugula
- ✓ 1 tbsp lemon
- ✓ 1/2 cup tahini sauce
- ✓ 12 falafels
- ✓ One sliced red onion
- ✓ 1/2 cup tabbouleh salad
- ✓ Three sprigs mint

Directions:

- ❖ Spread tahini sauce followed by the addition of arugula and crushed falafels over pita bread.
- ❖ Add tabbouleh salad, mint, and onions over pita and drizzle lemon juice.
- ❖ Wrap the pita bread and serve.

354) EASY ROASTED TOMATO AND BASIL SOUP

Preparation Time: 10 minutes	Cooking Time: 50 minutes	Servings: 6

Ingredients:

- ✓ 3 lb halved Roma tomatoes
- ✓ Olive oil
- ✓ Two chopped carrots
- ✓ Salt to taste
- ✓ Two chopped yellow onions
- ✓ Black pepper to taste
- ✓ Five minced garlic cloves
- ✓ 2 oz basil leaves
- ✓ 1 cup crushed tomatoes
- ✓ Three thyme sprigs
- ✓ 1 tsp dry oregano
- ✓ 2 tsp thyme leaves
- ✓ ½ tsp paprika
- ✓ 2.5 cups water
- ✓ ½ tsp cumin
- ✓ 1 tbsp lime juice

Directions:

- ❖ Mix salt, olive oil, carrot, black pepper, and tomatoes in a bowl.
- ❖ Transfer carrot mixture to a baking tray and bake in a preheated oven at 450 degrees for 30 minutes.
- ❖ Blend baked tomato mixture in a blender. You can use a little water if needed during blending.
- ❖ Sauté onions in heated olive oil over medium flame in a pot for three minutes.
- ❖ Mix garlic and cook for one more minute.
- ❖ Transfer the blended tomato mixture to the pot, followed by the addition of crushed tomatoes, water, spices, thyme, salt, basil, and pepper.
- ❖ Let it boil. Reduce the flame and simmer for 20 minutes.
- ❖ Drizzle lemon juice and serve.

355) GREEK-STYLE BLACK-EYED PEAS STEW

Preparation Time: 5 minutes	Cooking Time: 55 minutes	Servings: 6

Ingredients:

- Olive oil
- Four chopped garlic cloves
- 30 oz black-eyed peas
- One chopped yellow onion
- One chopped green bell pepper
- 15 oz diced tomato
- Three chopped carrots
- 1.5 tsp cumin
- One dry bay leaf
- 1 tsp dry oregano
- Kosher salt to taste
- ½ tsp red pepper flakes
- ½ tsp paprika
- Black pepper to taste
- 1 cup chopped parsley
- 1 tbsp of lime juice
- 2 cups of water

Directions:

- Cook garlic and onions in a heated oven in a Dutch oven over medium flame for five minutes with constant stirring.
- Stir in tomatoes, pepper, water, spices, bay leaf, and salt.
- Let it boil.
- Mix black-eyed beans and cook for five more minutes.
- Cover the oven and reduce the flame. Simmer for 30 minutes.
- Squeeze lemon juice and mix.
- Serve and enjoy.

356) GREEK CHICKEN GYROS WITH TZATZIKI SAUCE

Preparation Time: 10 minutes	Cooking Time: 8 minutes	Servings: 4

Ingredients:

- Greek Chicken
- 1 tbsp lemon juice
- 1/2 cup plain yogurt
- 1.25 tsp Italian-spiced salt
- 2 tbsp extra-virgin olive oil
- 1 cup Tzatziki sauce
- Four slices of pita bread
- Four chopped tomatoes
- 1/4 sliced red onion
- Tzatziki Sauce
- ½ halved cucumber
- ¾ cup Greek yogurt
- Two minced garlic cloves
- 1 tbsp red wine vinegar
- 1 tbsp chopped dill
- One pinch of kosher salt
- One pinch of black pepper

Directions:

- Marinate the chicken by mixing it with lemon juice, salt, and yogurt. Set aside for one hour.
- Heat olive oil in a skillet over medium flame.
- Add chicken without marinade and cook for five minutes from both sides. Transfer the cooked brown chicken to the plate.
- Mix all the ingredients of Tzatziki sauce in a bowl and set aside. The Tzatziki sauce is ready.
- Toast pita bread and place Tzatziki sauce, tomatoes, onions, and chicken pieces over pita bread. Wrap and serve.

Nutrition: Calories: 411 kcal Fat: 21 g Protein: 44 g Carbs: 10 g Fiber: 1 g

357) GREEK-STYLE CHICKEN MARINADE

Preparation Time: 5 minutes	Cooking Time: 15 minutes	Servings: 4

Ingredients:

- ✓ 1 lb boneless chicken breasts
- ✓ ¼ cup olive oil
- ✓ ½ tsp black pepper
- ✓ 1/3 cup Greek yogurt
- ✓ Four lemons
- ✓ 2 tbsp dried oregano
- ✓ Five minced garlic cloves
- ✓ 1 tsp kosher salt

Directions:

- ❖ Mix all the ingredients in a bowl and set aside for three hours.
- ❖ Preheat the grill and grill chicken and lemon slices for 20 minutes from both sides.
- ❖ Slice the grilled chicken and serve.

Nutrition: Calories: 304 kcal Fat: 19 g Protein: 25 g Carbs: 14 g Fiber: 4 g

358) ITALIAN STYLE CHICKEN QUINOA BOWL WITH BROCCOLI AND TOMATO

Preparation Time: 10 minutes	Cooking Time: 30 minutes	Servings: 3

Ingredients:

- ✓ Chicken
- ✓ 6 oz boneless chicken breast
- ✓ 1 cup Easy Roasted Feta and Broccoli
- ✓ 1/2 cup olive oil
- ✓ 1/2 tsp kosher salt
- ✓ Zest of one lemon
- ✓ 2 tsp dried oregano
- ✓ 1.5 tbsp lemon juice
- ✓ 1/4 tsp black pepper
- ✓ Two minced garlic cloves
- ✓ 1/2 cup Easy Roasted Tomatoes
- ✓ Quinoa
- ✓ 1 tsp kosher salt
- ✓ 1 cup dried quinoa
- ✓ Feta cheese to taste

Directions:

- ❖ Mix lemon juice, oregano, salt, olive oil, garlic, lemon zest, and pepper in a bowl.
- ❖ Add chicken and toss well. Set aside for one hour.
- ❖ Cook chicken in heat olive oil over medium flame for 15 minutes.
- ❖ Lower the flame and stir in tomatoes and broccoli and cook. Set aside.
- ❖ Add water and salt to a pot and bring it to a boil.
- ❖ Add quinoa and cook for ten minutes.
- ❖ Drain the quinoa and set aside.
- ❖ Add quinoa in a bowl, followed by the addition of chicken and veggies. Sprinkle salt, cheese, oil, and pepper.
- ❖ Serve and enjoy it.

Nutrition: Calories: 481 kcal Fat: 23 g Protein: 24 g Carbs: 45 g Fiber: 7 g

359) EASY CHICKEN PICCATA

Preparation Time: 10 minutes	Cooking Time: 10 minutes	Servings: 4

Ingredients:

- ✓ 1.5 lb boneless chicken breasts
- ✓ One lemon
- ✓ 2 tbsp canola oil
- ✓ 1 tsp kosher salt
- ✓ 1 cup chicken broth
- ✓ 1 tsp black pepper
- ✓ 2 tbsp capers
- ✓ 3 tbsp butter
- ✓ 1/3 cup all-purpose flour

Directions:

- ❖ Mix salt, flour, and pepper in a bowl. Coat chicken with the flour mixture. Set aside.
- ❖ Cook chicken pieces in heated butter and canola oil over medium flame for five minutes from both sides. Shift cooked pieces onto the plate.
- ❖ Lower the flame and pour broth and add sliced lemon, butter (1 tbsp), lemon juice, capers, and cook for five minutes.
- ❖ Pour the sauce over chicken pieces and serve with cauliflower or noodles.

Nutrition: Calories: 381 kcal Fat: 20 g Protein: 37 g Carbs: 11 g Fiber: 1 g

360) ITALIAN CHOPPED GRILLED VEGETABLE WITH FARRO

Preparation Time: 5 minutes	Cooking Time: 50 minutes	Servings: 2

Ingredients:

- ✓ 1 cup dried farro
- ✓ 1 Portobello mushroom
- ✓ 3 cups vegetable broth
- ✓ One sliced red bell pepper
- ✓ 1/2 sliced red onion
- ✓ 8 oz asparagus
- ✓ One sliced zucchini
- ✓ Olive oil as required
- ✓ 1/4 cup halved Kalamata olives
- ✓ One sliced yellow squash
- ✓ Kosher salt to taste
- ✓ 1-pint Greek yogurt
- ✓ Black pepper to taste
- ✓ 2 tbsp minced cucumber
- ✓ One chopped garlic clove
- ✓ 1 tbsp lemon juice
- ✓ 1 tsp chopped dill
- ✓ 1 tsp chopped mint
- ✓ Red bell pepper hummus
- ✓ 1/8 cup feta cheese

Directions:

- ❖ In a large pot, add broth and farro. Let it boil over a high flame.
- ❖ Lower the flame to medium and cook for half an hour with occasional stirring.
- ❖ Mix veggies with salt, olive oil, and pepper.
- ❖ Grill the veggies in a preheated grill until marks appear on them. Keep them aside.
- ❖ Whisk cucumber, salt, mint, dill, yogurt, lemon juice, and garlic in a bowl.
- ❖ Make the layers of farro, grilled veggies, hummus, olives, and cheese.
- ❖ Pour yogurt sauce and sprinkle mint and serve.

Nutrition: Calories: 140 kcal Fat: 6 g Protein: 4 g Carbs: 20 g Fiber: 5 g

361) QUICK PORK ESCALOPES IN 30 MINUTES WITH LEMONS AND CAPERS

Preparation Time: 10 minutes	Cooking Time: 20 minutes	Servings: 4

Ingredients:

- ✓ Four boneless pork chops
- ✓ 1/4 cup all-purpose flour
- ✓ Eight sage leaves
- ✓ kosher salt to taste
- ✓ 2 tbsp chopped parsley
- ✓ 4 tbsp butter
- ✓ Black pepper to taste
- ✓ 1 tbsp vegetable oil
- ✓ 1/4 cup capers
- ✓ 1/2 cup white wine
- ✓ 1 cup chicken stock
- ✓ One sliced lemon
- ✓ 4 tbsp lemon juice

Directions:

- ❖ One each pork chops, place two sage leaves on both sides. Set aside.
- ❖ In a bowl, whisk salt, flour, and pepper.
- ❖ Coat pork chops with flour. Keep the sage leaves in place.
- ❖ Melt butter in a skillet over medium flame.
- ❖ Cook pork chops for five minutes from both sides.
- ❖ Clean the skillet and melt butter in it.
- ❖ Pour wine and add capers in skillet. Cook to concentrate the wine.
- ❖ Pour stock, lemon slices, and lemon juice. Let it boil for five more minutes.
- ❖ Place pork in sauce and cook for two minutes.
- ❖ Sprinkle parsley and serve.

Nutrition: Calories: 415 kcal Fat: 7 g Protein: 31 g Carbs: 14 g Fiber: 8 g

362) GREEK-STYLE CHICKEN KEBABS

Preparation Time: 40 minutes	Cooking Time: 15 minutes	Servings: 6

Ingredients:

- ✓ 1 lb boneless chicken breasts
- ✓ 1/4 cup olive oil
- ✓ One sliced red bell pepper
- ✓ 1/3 cup Greek yogurt
- ✓ 10 tbsp lemons juice
- ✓ Four chopped garlic cloves
- ✓ Zest of one lemon
- ✓ 2 tbsp dried oregano
- ✓ 1/2 tsp black pepper
- ✓ One sliced zucchini
- ✓ 1 tsp kosher salt
- ✓ One sliced red onion

Directions:

- ❖ Whisk all the ingredients except chicken in a bowl. Add chicken and toss to coat chicken evenly. Set aside four hours for better results.
- ❖ Thread chicken, zucchini, onion, and bell pepper on the skewers.
- ❖ Grill the chicken, skewers on a preheated grill for 15 minutes, occasionally turning and basting with marinade.

Nutrition: Calories: 224 kcal Fat: 13 g Protein: 18 g Carbs: 13 g Fiber: 4 g

363) EASY PASTA WITH SHRIMP AND ROASTED RED PEPPERS AND ARTICHOKES

Preparation Time: 10 minutes	Cooking Time: 25 minutes	Servings: 8

Ingredients:

- ✓ 12 oz farfalle pasta
- ✓ 1/4 cup butter
- ✓ 1.5 lb shrimp
- ✓ Three chopped garlic cloves
- ✓ 1 cup sliced artichoke hearts
- ✓ 12 oz roasted and chopped red bell peppers
- ✓ 1/2 cup dry white wine
- ✓ 1/4 cup basil
- ✓ 1/2 cup whipping cream
- ✓ 3 tbsp drained capers
- ✓ 1 tsp grated lemon peel
- ✓ 3/4 cup feta cheese
- ✓ 2 tbsp lemon juice
- ✓ 2 oz toasted pine nuts

Directions:

- ❖ Boil water in a pot and cook pasta in it.
- ❖ Drain pasta and set aside.
- ❖ Melt butter in a skillet over medium flame. Sauté garlic and cook for one minute.
- ❖ Stir in shrimps and cook for about two minutes.
- ❖ Mix artichokes, capers, bell pepper, and wine. Let it boil.
- ❖ Lower the flame and let it simmer for two minutes with occasional stirring.
- ❖ Add whipping cream, lemon juice, and lemon zest.
- ❖ Let it boil for five minutes.
- ❖ Transfer the cooked shrimps over pasta and mix well.
- ❖ Spread cheese, basil, and nuts and serve.

Nutrition: Calories: 627 kcal Fat: 24 g Protein: 38 g Carbs: 58 g Fiber: 3 g

364) CHICKEN CAPRESE QUICK IN 30 MINUTES

Preparation Time: 10 minutes	Cooking Time: 20 minutes	Servings: 4

Ingredients:

- ✓ Two boneless chicken breasts
- ✓ Black pepper to taste
- ✓ 1 tbsp butter
- ✓ 1 tbsp extra virgin olive oil
- ✓ 6 oz Pesto
- ✓ Eight chopped tomatoes
- ✓ Six grated mozzarella cheese
- ✓ Balsamic glaze as needed
- ✓ Kosher salt to taste
- ✓ Basil as required

Directions:

- ❖ Mix salt, sliced chicken, and pepper in a bowl. Set aside for ten minutes.
- ❖ Melt butter in a skillet over medium flame.
- ❖ Cook chicken pieces in melted butter for five minutes from both sides.
- ❖ Remove from the flame. Sprinkle pesto and place mozzarella cheese and tomatoes over chicken pieces.
- ❖ Bake in a preheated oven at 400 degrees for 12 minutes.
- ❖ Garnish with balsamic glaze and serve.

Nutrition: Calories: 232 kcal Fat: 15 g Protein: 18 g Carbs: 5 g Fiber: 1 g

365) SPECIAL GRILLED LEMON CHICKEN SKEWERS

Preparation Time: 10 minutes	Cooking Time: 10 minutes	Servings: 6

Ingredients:

- ✓ Two boneless chicken breasts
- ✓ Seven green onions
- ✓ Four minced garlic cloves
- ✓ Three lemons
- ✓ 1 tbsp dried oregano
- ✓ 1 tsp kosher salt
- ✓ 1/4 cup olive oil
- ✓ 1/2 tsp black pepper

Directions:

- ❖ Whisk salt, lemon juice, olive oil, garlic, lemon zest, black pepper, oregano, and sliced chicken pieces in a bowl. Set aside for four hours.
- ❖ Thread chicken, onions, and lemon slices onto the skewer.
- ❖ Grill chicken skewers for 15 minutes on preheated grill over medium flames with often turning.
- ❖ Serve when chicken is fully cooked.

366) TASTY JUICY SALMON BURGERS

Preparation Time: 10 minutes	Cooking Time: 4 minutes	Servings: 4

Ingredients:

- ✓ 1.5 lb sliced salmon fillet
- ✓ 3 tbsp minced green onions
- ✓ 1 tsp coriander
- ✓ 2 tsp Dijon mustard
- ✓ 1/3 cup bread crumbs
- ✓ 1 tsp sumac
- ✓ 1 cup chopped parsley
- ✓ ½ tsp sweet paprika
- ✓ Kosher Salt to taste
- ✓ ¼ cup olive oil
- ✓ ½ tsp black pepper
- ✓ One lemon
- ✓ Toppings
- ✓ One sliced red onion
- ✓ Tzatziki Sauce
- ✓ One sliced tomato
- ✓ 6 oz baby arugula

Directions:

- ❖ Blend mustard and salmon in a blender.
- ❖ Shift the mixture in a container. Add all the spices, parsley, salt, and onions. Mix well and set aside for 30 minutes.
- ❖ Make patties out of salmon mixture and place in a tray.
- ❖ Coat all the patties with bread crumbs from both sides.
- ❖ Fry the patties in heated olive oil over medium flame for five minutes each from both sides.
- ❖ Drizzle lemon juice over the cooked patties.
- ❖ Spread Tzatziki sauce over the bun, followed by the layer of salmon, arugula, onions, and tomatoes. The salmon burgers are ready. Serve and enjoy it.

367) SPECIAL BRAISED EGGPLANT AND CHICKPEAS

Preparation Time: 20 minutes	Cooking Time: 55 minutes	Servings: 6

Ingredients:

- ✓ 1.5 lb chopped eggplant
- ✓ Olive Oil
- ✓ Kosher salt
- ✓ One chopped yellow onion
- ✓ One chopped carrot
- ✓ One diced green bell pepper
- ✓ Six minced garlic cloves
- ✓ 1.5 tsp sweet paprika
- ✓ Two dry bay leaves
- ✓ 1 tsp organic coriander
- ✓ ¾ tsp cinnamon
- ✓ 1 tsp dry oregano
- ✓ ½ tsp organic turmeric
- ✓ 28 oz chopped tomato
- ✓ ½ tsp black pepper
- ✓ 30 oz chickpeas
- ✓ Handful parsley and mint for garnishing

Directions:

- ❖ Sauté onions, carrots, and bell peppers in heated olive oil over medium flame for four minutes with constant stirring.
- ❖ Stir in salt, bay leaf, garlic, and spices and cook for one minute.
- ❖ Mix eggplant, chickpeas, tomato, and chickpea liquid.
- ❖ Let it boil for ten minutes.
- ❖ Remove the pan from flame and cover.
- ❖ Now, bake in a preheated oven at 400 degrees for 45 minutes.
- ❖ Sprinkle herbs and serve with any sauce.

Nutrition: Calories: 240 kcal Fat: 5.1 g Protein: 10.6 g Carbs: 42 g Fiber: 15 g

368) ITALIAN STYLE TUNA SALAD SANDWICHES

Preparation Time: 5 minutes	Cooking Time: 0 minute	Servings: 4

Ingredients:

- ✓ 4 tsp red wine vinegar
- ✓ 4 tsp olive oil
- ✓ Eight bread slices
- ✓ ¼ cup chopped red onion
- ✓ 1/3 cup chopped sun-dried tomatoes
- ✓ ¼ tsp black pepper
- ✓ ¼ cup sliced olives
- ✓ 3 tbsp mayonnaise
- ✓ 2 tsp capers
- ✓ Four lettuce leaves
- ✓ 12 oz tuna

Directions:

- ❖ Mix wine and olive oil.
- ❖ Brush bread from both sides with oil mixture.
- ❖ Mix all the ingredients except lettuce and bread slices in a bowl.
- ❖ Place lettuce on each bread slices brushed with oil. Spread tuna mixture and cover with second bread piece and serve.

Nutrition: Calories: 293 kcal Fat: 10 g Protein: 21.2 g Carbs: 31.3 g Fiber: 4.6 g

369)   MOROCCAN-STYLE VEGETABLE TAGINE

Preparation Time: 15 minutes	Cooking Time: 40 minutes	Servings: 5

Ingredients:

- ¼ cup extra virgin olive oil
- Ten chopped garlic cloves
- Two chopped yellow onions
- Two chopped carrots
- One sliced sweet potato
- Two sliced potatoes
- Salt
- 1 tsp coriander
- 1 tbsp Harissa spice
- 1 tsp cinnamon
- 2 cups tomatoes
- ½ tsp turmeric
- ½ cup chopped dried apricot
- 2 cups cooked chickpeas
- Handful fresh parsley leaves
- ½ cup vegetable broth
- 1 tbsp lemon juice

Directions:

- Sauté onions in heated olive oil at high flame for five minutes in a Dutch oven.
- Stir in veggies, salt, garlic, and spices. Mix well and cook for eight minutes over medium flame with constant stirring.
- Mix in broth, apricot, and tomatoes and cook for the next ten minutes.
- Reduce the flame and let it simmer for 25 minutes.
- Add chickpeas and cook for five minutes.
- Sprinkle parsley and lemon juice and mix well.
- Serve and enjoy it.

Nutrition: Calories: 448 kcal Fat: 18.4 g Protein: 16.9 g Carbs: 60.7 g Fiber: 24 g

370)   ITALIAN-STYLE GRILLED BALSAMIC CHICKEN WITH OLIVE TAPENADE

Preparation Time: 10 minutes	Cooking Time: 30 minutes	Servings: 2

Ingredients:

- Two boneless chicken breasts
- 1/4 cup olive oil
- 1/4 cup balsamic vinegar
- 1/8 cup garlic mustard
- 1.5 tbsp balsamic vinegar
- Three minced garlic cloves
- 1 tbsp lemon juice
- 1 tbsp chopped herbs of choice
- 1 tsp kosher salt
- 1/2 tsp black pepper

Directions:

- Combine garlic, balsamic vinegar, lemon juice, pepper, olive oil, herbs, salt, and mustard in a bowl. Add chicken and toss well to coat chicken.
- Set aside for three hours.
- Brush oil over chicken pieces and grill gates.
- Cook chicken on grill gates for ten minutes from both sides.
- Occasionally brush the chicken with marinade while grilling it.
- When marks appear over the chicken, shift the chicken to the grill gate's cooler side and cook there for 12 minutes.
- Again, shift the chicken to the heated side of the grill gate and cook for ten more minutes.
- Place the grilled chicken on a plate and cover to keep it warm.
- Serve and enjoy it.

Nutrition: Calories: 352 kcal Fat: 21 g Protein: 35 mg Carbs: 5 g Fiber: 1 g

371)	ITALIAN LINGUINE AND ZUCCHINI NOODLES WITH SHRIMP	
Preparation Time: 20 minutes	**Cooking Time:** 20 minutes	**Servings:** 6

Ingredients:

- ✓ 2/3 cup extra virgin olive oil
- ✓ 1 lb shrimp
- ✓ Four minced garlic cloves
- ✓ Black pepper to taste
- ✓ 12 oz wheat linguine
- ✓ kosher salt to taste

- ✓ 3 tbsp butter
- ✓ Three zucchinis
- ✓ One lemon zested
- ✓ 1 tsp red chili flakes
- ✓ 3 tbsp lemon juice
- ✓ A handful of chopped parsley
- ✓ 1/2 cup shredded Parmesan cheese

Directions:

- ❖ Add salt, garlic, shrimps, pepper, and olive oil. Toss well to coat evenly. Keep it aside.
- ❖ Pour water into a pot and add salt to it. Let it boil and cook linguine in boiling water. Drain linguine and set aside.
- ❖ Heat olive oil in a skillet over medium heat and cook shrimps in it for three minutes from both sides. Shift the cooked shrimps into the plate.
- ❖ Melt butter in the same pan and sauté garlic, lemon juice, chili flakes, and lemon zest for one minute.
- ❖ Pour in pasta water in another pan and cook for three minutes. Add zucchini noodles and cook for two minutes with constant stirring.
- ❖ Transfer the noodles to the garlic mixture pan. Add linguine and cheese. Toss well.
- ❖ Pour in more of the pasta water to make a sauce of the desired level.
- ❖ Add shrimp, zucchini, salt, and pepper, and mix well.
- ❖ You can spread more cheese if you like.
- ❖ Garnish with parsley and serve.

Nutrition: Calories: 521 kcal Fat: 22 g Protein: 28 g Carbs: 52 g Fiber: 4 g

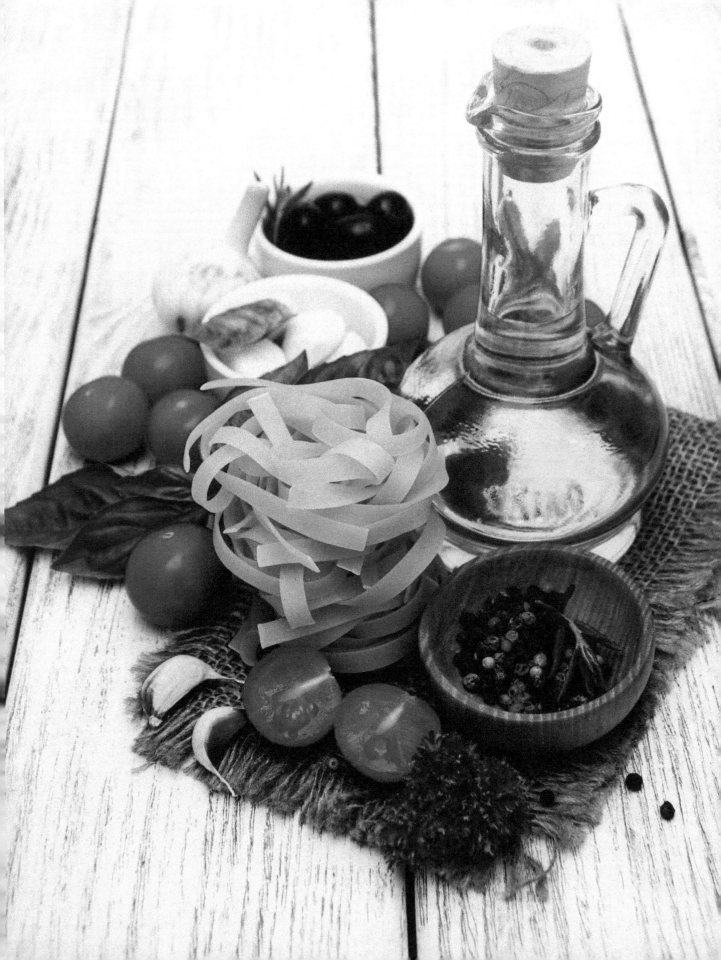

Bibliography

FROM THE SAME AUTHOR

ITALIAN COOKBOOK FOR ONE - More than 120 Very Easy Recipes for Beginners! Delight yourself like in a restaurant with the best meals for weight loss and heart health!

ITALIAN DIET FOR BEGINNERS *Cookbook* - 120+ Super Easy Recipes to Start a Healthier Lifestyle! Discover the tastiest Diet overall to lose weight and stay Healthy!

ITALIAN DIET FOR MEN *Cookbook* - More than 120 seafood, vegetarian and meat recipes from the Best Mediterranean Cuisine! Stay FIT and HEALTHY with the perfect diet to lose weight before summer!

ITALIAN DIET FOR WOMEN *Cookbook* - The Best 120+ recipes for weight loss and stay HEALTHY! Maintain FIT your body and delight yourself with the best diet overall for heart health!

ITALIAN DIET FOR KIDS *Cookbook* - The Most Delicious 120 Recipes for Children, tested BY Kids FOR Kids! Stay FIT and HEALTHY with many seafood and vegetarian meals, HAVING FUN as in a restaurant!

ITALIAN COOKBOOK FOR TWO - The Best 220+ Seafood and Vegetarian Recipes For Mum and Kids! Stay HEALTHY and lose weight preparing these delicious meals with your family!

ITALIAN COOKBOOK FOR COUPLE - 220+ Delicious Recipes to make together! Eat with your Partner as in a Restaurant with the most complete guide about the Italian Cuisine for two!

ITALIAN COOKBOOK FOR BEGINNER CHEF - More than 220 Very Easy Recipes to Start your Italian Restaurant Cuisine! Delight yourself and your Friends with the Best Mediterranean Meals like a Chef!

ITALIAN COOKBOOK FOR MEDITERRANEAN ATHLETES - The Best 220+ Seafood and Vegetarian Recipes for Weight Loss and Heart Health! Stay FIT and LIGHT with The Most Delicious Diet Overall!

ITALIAN COOKBOOK FOR WEIGHT LOSS Cookbook - More than 300 HEALTHY Mediterranean Recipes For Weight Loss and stay FIT! Tone your Body before SUMMER and Maintain your Perfect Weight with The Best Diet Overall!

THE COMPLETE ITALIAN DIET Cookbook - The Best 320+ Super Easy Recipes to Start your Perfect HEALTHY Lifestyle! Discover the Italian Cuisine with the Tastiest and Healthiest Recipes!

ITALIAN AND MEDITERRANEAN DIET FOR FAMILY Cookbook - More than 300 Seafood and Vegetarian Recipes For Mum, Dad and Kids! Stay HEALTHY and HAPPY as in a Restaurant preparing these delicious meals with your family!

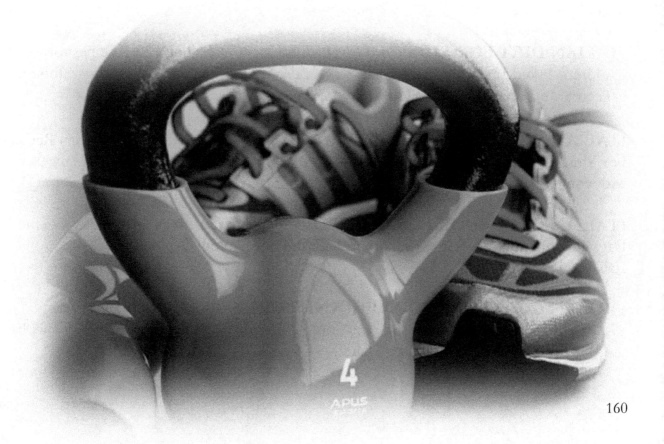

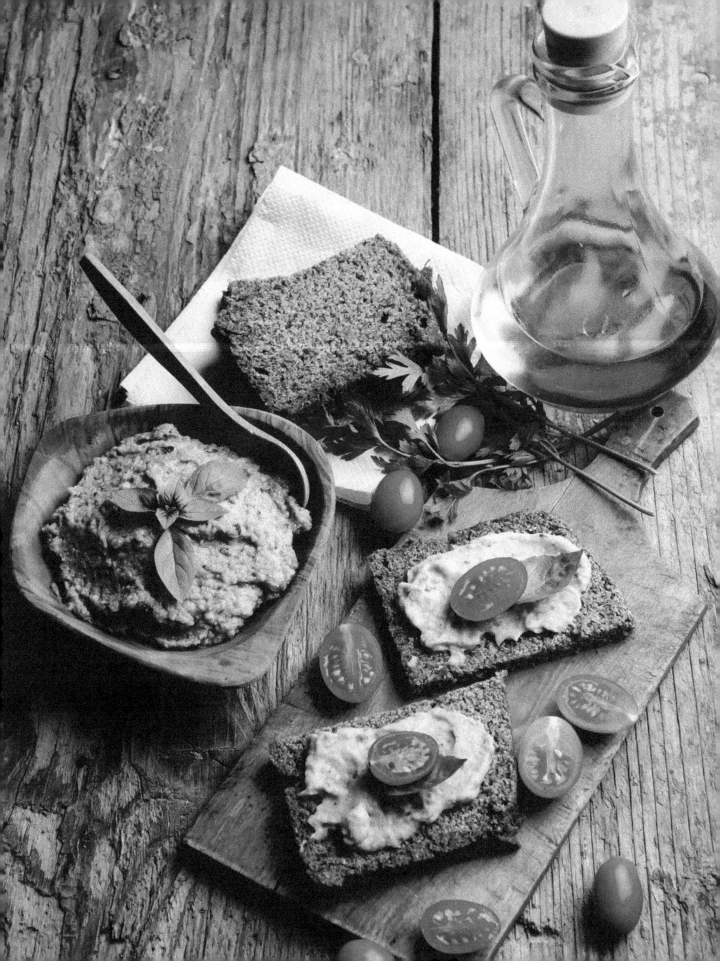

Conclusion

Thanks for reading "Italian Diet for Weight loss *Cookbook*"!

I hope you liked this Cookbook!

I wish you to achieve all your goals!

Olivia Rossi

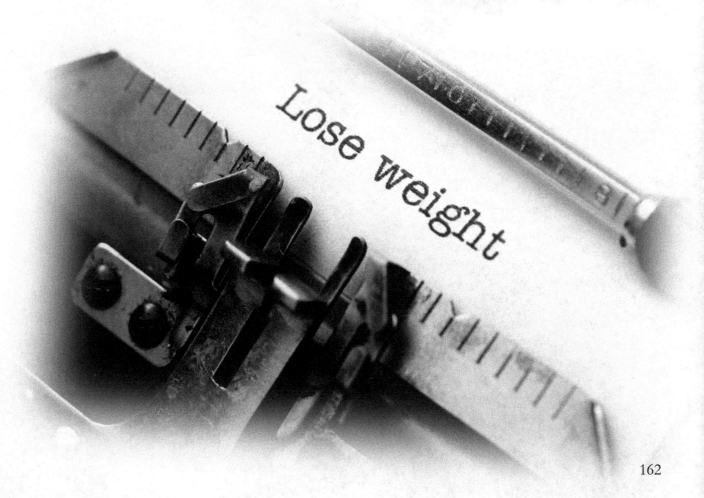